Fluid Therapy in C

T.L. CHAMBERS

FRCP, FRCPE
Physician to the Children's Department
Southmead Hospital, Bristol
and to the Bristol Royal
Hospital for Sick Children
Clinical Lecturer in Child Health
University of Bristol

*With a Chapter
on the Burned Child by*

R.W. GRIFFITHS

MS, FRCS
Consultant Plastic Surgeon
Northern General Hospital
Sheffield

Blackwell Scientific Publications

OXFORD LONDON EDINBURGH
BOSTON PALO ALTO MELBOURNE

To all
my parents

First published 1987

Set by BH Typesetters & Designers
Oxfordshire

Printed and bound in Great Britain
by Billing & Sons Ltd, Worcester

DISTRIBUTORS

USA
    Year Book Medical Publishers,
    35 East Wacker Drive,
    Chicago, Illinois 60601

Canada
    The C.V. Mosby Company,
    5240 Finch Avenue East,
    Scarborough, Ontario

Australia
    Blackwell Scientific Publications
    (Australia) Pty Ltd,
    107 Barry Street,
    Carlton, Victoria 3053

British Library
Cataloguing in Publication Data

Chambers, T.L.
    Fluid therapy in childhood.
    1. Water-electrolyte inbalances
    in children
    I. Title   II. Griffiths, R.W.
    618.92'39   RJ399.W35

ISBN 0 632 00899 7

Contents

Preface

Authors of books on fluid therapy have to be careful that the result resembles neither an attenuated textbook of paediatrics nor a cookery book. Water and electrolyte management is essentially practical and is best learned by dealing with individual patients under the friendly eye of a more experienced colleague. Practical techniques are certainly best learned this way and I have not described them here. This book should be read over a cup of coffee whilst waiting for laboratory results or watching an ill patient.

Bristol 1986   T.L. Chambers

Acknowledgements

I am grateful to Mr Griffiths for his chapter on the burned child and to my colleagues Dr D. Burman, Dr M.D.C. Donaldson and Dr G. Walters for reading the manuscript and offering comments and criticisms — although, of course, the responsibility for its accuracy is mine. Miss J.D. Hamblin typed most of the script that Mr Peter Saugman of Blackwell Scientific Publications persuasively encouraged me to complete.

Theoretical Background

1

Basic Physiology

General

It is important to know about underlying physiological principles before attempting to solve clinical and theoretical problems of water and electrolyte balance in children. Some aspects are not fully understood, mainly because of limitations of research in children; in these cases reasonable assumptions may be made. Physiological changes at birth, somatic growth and differences in body proportions each impose their own complexities on fluid balance in children.

Units and terminology

In many parts of the world metric SI (Systeme Internationale) units have replaced the fractional centimetre, gram and second units. The basic SI unit for volume is the cubic metre (m^3), but as this is too large for everyday use the cubic decimetre (dm^3) or decilitre (dl) is used. Amounts of substances are expressed as moles (mol) and millimoles (mmol), and the concentration of a substance in solution is expressed in millimoles $(10^{-3}$ mol) or micromoles $(10^{-6}$ mol) per litre (mmol = mg/molecular weight).

SI units also replace the equivalency terminology based upon the combining power of substances, as it is now recognized that the number of molecules present is of greater physiological importance. This is particularly so when considering fluid shifts; the direction of such shifts is determined by the number of particles present in the fluid compartments (osmotic pressure) rather than their weight or electronic properties. Thus the units (milli)mole and (milli)osmole are interchangeable. All particles in solution, whether ionized or not, constitute the total solute, and the value of this total is expressed as the number of milliosmoles. If this total is added to water to make a total volume of 1 litre the resulting solute concentration is the *osmolarity* (normal osmolarity of plasma is about 300 mmol/l). If the total solute is added to 1 litre, that is 1 kg, of water the concentration is the *osmolality* (plasma osmolality is *c.* 285 mmol/kg). Osmolality is the term that will be used in this book.

3

Fluid compartments

The sum of all the fluids in the body except the lumen of the gut and urinary tract is the total body water (TBW). In the newborn this constitutes about 80% body weight, and from a year onwards about 60% body weight (Table 1.1). These relationships are influenced by body build; fat cells contain little water so the TBW of an obese child will be a smaller fraction of the body weight than in a normal or lean child. TBW is divided into water inside cells, intracellular fluid (ICF), and water outside cells, extracellular fluid (ECF). ECF is further distributed between the intravascular fluid or blood volume and extravascular or interstitial fluid. A small amount (1–2%) ECF, called transcellular fluid, represents cerebrospinal, ocular, synovial and other lubricant fluids. The relationships of the fluid volumes are shown in Figure 1.1.

Table 1.1   Total body water as percentage of body weight (BW) at various ages

Age	% BW
12-week foetus	90
Newborn	80
12 months	60
Adult	60

Extracellular fluid

Quantity

This changes considerably during foetal and postnatal life as shown in Table 1.2; the most abrupt changes take place immediately after birth. After adolescence boys have more body water than girls, who possess more body fat.

Quality, the anion gap and pseudohyponatraemia

The distribution of solutes in the blood compartments of ECF are shown in Figure 1.2; interstitial fluid contains more chloride and less protein than plasma and its osmolality is theoretically lower.

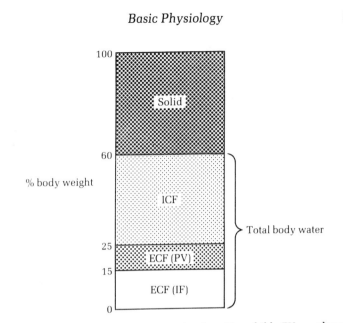

Figure 1.1 The fluid compartments in the older child. PV = plasma volume (including transcellular and bone water); IF = interstitial fluid.

Table 1.2   ECF as percentage of body weight at various ages

Age	% BW
28-week foetus	55
Newborn	40
12 months	25
Adult	20

The greater hydrostatic pressure of the vascular system prevents the transfer of water from interstices to plasma.

If the values of sodium, chloride and bicarbonate in plasma are examined the following relation is demonstrated: $Na^+ + K^+ = Cl^- + HCO_3^- + c.\ 15$ (e.g. 138 mmol/l + 4 mmol/l = 105 mmol/l + 23 mmol/l + 14 mmol/l). This extra 14 mmol/l, the anion gap, represents unmeasured protein, sulphate, phosphate and other ions. A larger (> 20 mmol/l) gap suggests the presence of some additional anion, such as in salicylate poisoning, lactic acidosis or in diabetic ketoacidosis (acetoacetate).

The osmolality of the extracellular fluid is maintained at 280–290 mmol/kg by controls which will be discussed later. Sodium is the most important cation in the ECF contributing to plasma osmolality, and an approximate value for plasma osmolality can be obtained from the plasma level of sodium: plasma osmolality (mmol/kg) = 2 × plasma Na (mmol/l). In the presence of elevated levels of urea or glucose the following correction will be required: plasma osmolality = 2 × Na (mmol/l) + plasma glucose (mmol/l) + plasma urea (mmol/l).

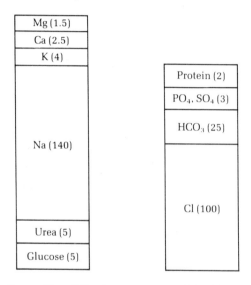

Figure 1.2   Composition of blood compartments of the ECF (in mmol/l).

Furthermore, if the plasma contains excess lipid, such as in nephrotic syndrome or diabetic ketoacidosis, the measured plasma sodium may be falsely low. The reason for this is that the plasma sodium is measured in mmol per litre of plasma which contains water and solute in the aqueous phase and lipid dispersed throughout. Electrolyte values are expressed as mmol per litre of *whole* plasma, and if there is significant lipaemia plasma water will be displaced and the plasma sodium lowered (see Figure 1.3). This decrease is artefactual as the sodium concentration in plasma water remains the same. If there is doubt about the contribution that lipaemia is making to hyponatraemia then a depression of freezing point method should be used to measure plasma osmolality, which roughly reflects the sodium content of plasma water only. Modern ion-selective electrodes will measure the true plasma sodium level. Pseudohyponatraemia needs no treatment in itself as it will improve with correction of the primary cause; indeed aggressive 'correction' of this artefactual level may be disastrous.

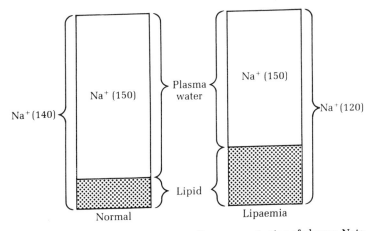

Figure 1.3 Influence of lipaemia on sodium concentration of plasma. Note that the concentration of Na^+ per litre of plasma water is constant, but that the concentration of Na^+ per litre of whole plasma will vary with the amount of lipid present.

Intracellular fluid

Access to ICF is difficult and therefore less is known about its composition and function than ECF. ICF is customarily represented as a homogeneous entity, whereas in fact its composition differs from cell to cell throughout the body.

Quantity

The relative volume of ICF is more stable with age than the ECF; at birth it is about 30% of body weight rising to 40% by one year.

Quality

The electrolyte composition is very different to that of ECF; the chief cations are potassium and magnesium, and there is very little sodium. Phosphate, proteins and, to a lesser extent, sulphate are the main intracellular anions; there is much less bicarbonate and negligible chloride (see Figure 1.4). The plasma and intracellular fluids are separated by a selectively permeable membrane through which sodium, potassium and chloride are freely diffuseable but

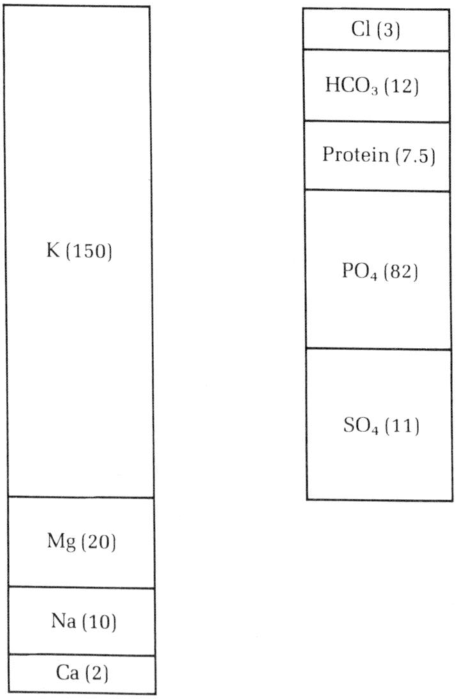

Figure 1.4 Electrolyte content of the ICF (in mmol/l).

protein is not. Regulation of ionic content is complex; the Donnan theory predicts that when two electrolyte solutions (such as ECF and ICF) are separated by a membrane which is permeable to some of the ions, the diffusable ions will tend to distribute themselves between the two compartments in similar proportions. However, this does not happen between the ICF and ECF because active transport mechanisms exist in the cell wall to preserve the relationship of electrolytes between the ICF and interstitial fluid, with potassium being retained within the cell and sodium pumped out.

Factors influencing fluid shifts

The composition of fluid compartments changes in health and disease according to outside influences, such as excessive fluid loss in diarrhoea or sweating from severe exercise. A number of processes exist to allow movement of water and solutes between compartments, tending to restore homeostasis.

Diffusion

This is the process by which molecules spread from a solution of high concentration to one of low concentration down a chemical gradient. Diffusion occurs within fluid compartments and between them through semipermeable membranes.

Osmosis

Solvent (water) molecules pass across a membrane impermeable to solute from a solution of low solute concentration to one of higher solute concentration (Figure 1.5A and B). This movement can be prevented by applying pressure to the concentrated solution; this is the osmotic pressure of the solution (Figure 1.5C). This pressure is proportional to the number of particles (mainly ions in the case of fluid compartments) in solution per kilogram of solvent, which is the osmolality of the solution. The osmolality of a solution such as an infusion fluid relative to plasma is known as tonicity. Isotonic fluid have the same osmolality as plasma; hyper- and hypotonic fluids have respectively greater or lesser osmotic pressures than plasma. Some fluids that are isotonic in infusion bags rapidly become hypotonic in the body because the solute is metabolized — for example 5% dextrose solutions.

Active transport

Some ions and non-ionized molecules are transported across cell membranes by carriers such as hormones (insulin). If this transport is down a concentration gradient, no energy is used. If the direction is from a low to a high concentration against a gradient, then energy is required from cell metabolism, usually ATP (adenosine triphosphate) dependent.

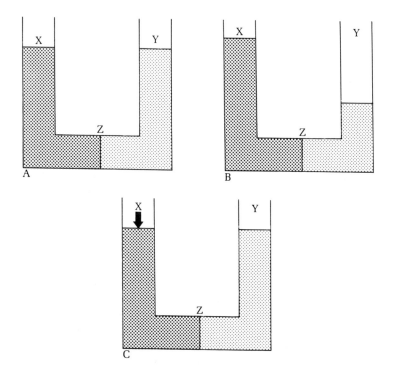

Figure 1.5 Osmotic movement of water molecules. A. The solution in X is hypertonic to Y, and Z is a semipermeable membrane. B. Water passes from Y to X through Z, to make solutions X and Y of similar concentration (isotonic). Note that: (1) the volume of solution is greater in limb X because of the fluid shift; and (2) the resulting solution in X is more dilute than at first, and the solution in Y is more concentrated. C. The pressure applied to limb X to prevent the movement of water from Y to X is the osmotic pressure.

2

Electrolytes and Water:
Controls and Balance

Sodium

Intake

The dietary sodium content varies widely throughout the world, and is also related to age. About 1-2 mmol sodium/kg/24 hours is regarded as the average intake required for growth and to balance losses in a healthy growing infant; adults ingest 75-150 mmol sodium/24 hours in an average diet. The sensation of salt loss is not so finely developed as thirst due to water loss; nevertheless in salt-losing states such as cystic fibrosis and salt-wasting nephropathy, salt craving may be experienced.

Distribution

Sodium is the principal cation in the ECF and plays an important part in maintaining the intravascular and interstitial fluid volumes. The total amount of sodium in the body is 60 mmol/kg body weight distributed throughout the various tissues (Table 2.1). The total exchangeable sodium in the body (outside the skeleton) is very much higher in the foetus compared with the adult; the difference is explained by the foetus possessing a proportionately larger volume of ECF.

Regulation and excretion

Small amounts of sodium are lost in sweat and faeces. Renal excretion is the most important regulator of total body sodium and its concentration in body fluids. Large amounts of sodium are filtered at the glomerulus under the influence of changes in renal bloodflow, glomerular capillary hydrostatic pressure, changes in plasma proteins, the permeability of the glomerulus, and the total number of glomeruli. Up to 99% is reabsorbed throughout the nephron, mainly in the proximal tubule along with chloride.

Table 2.1　Approximate distribution of body sodium

	BW (mmol/kg)	% of whole
ECF		
Plasma	6.5	10
Interstitial fluid	17	30
Connective tissue and cartilage	7	12
Bone	20	36
Transcellular	1.5	3
	52	91
ICF	6	9
Total	58	100

Smaller amounts are reabsorbed or exchanged for potassium and hydrogen ions (H^+) in the distal tubules, influenced by the concentration of protein (oncotic pressure) in the blood circulating through peritubular capillaries, by aldosterone (Figure 2.1) and other adrenal hormones, and, possibly, by further unidentified hormones. In severe sodium deficiency or reduced ECF volume the output may drop to 1 mmol/24 hours whilst outputs of 300+ mmol/24 hours may be produced by diets liberal in sodium. Control systems in the infant are well adapted to an intake of sodium corresponding to its concentration in human milk (7 mmol/l), but the lower glomerular filtration rate and limited tubular function of the infant mean that the response to great dietary variations of sodium intake are blunted, and sodium excess or deficit is more easily produced at this age.

Pathological states

An increased plasma sodium (hypernatraemia; Na $\geqslant$ 145 mmol/l) results either from diminished intake or excessive loss of water, or from excessive sodium intake. This may occur, for example, by the injudicious use of salt to induce emesis in poisons, its accidental addition to proprietary baby milks instead of sugar, or by deliberate poisoning. Hyponatraemia (Na < 130 mmol/l) is caused by an inadequate intake or excessive loss of salt, or an excessive intake of

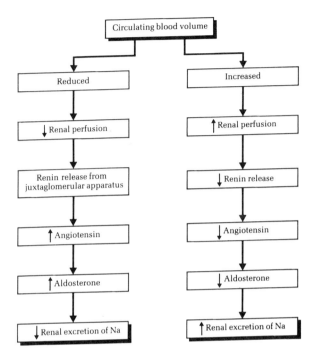

Figure 2.1 Influences on renal sodium handling. Note that other mediators such as atrial natiuretic factor may also be influential.

water. Hyponatraemia may occur, for example, with persistent vomiting or nasogastric suction when fluid loss is replaced as water, or when there is inappropriate secretion of antidiuretic hormone.

Plasma sodium concentration

This does not indicate the absolute amount of sodium in the plasma, and interpretation of its level must take into account the state of hydration of the child. Deviation from the normal may be caused by changes in sodium or water content; if the change is abrupt it usually reflects a change in body water which may be detected by changes in body weight. The plasma sodium may be used as a very approx-

Chapter 2

imate guide for repletion in deficiency states using the formula: sodium deficit = (135–z) × 0.3* × wt (kg), where z is the measured plasma sodium (but remember pseudohyponatraemia, see Figure 1.3).

Potassium

Intake

The requirement for potassium is similar to sodium, i.e. about 2 mmol/kg/24 hours, and is supplied to infants in milk. In older children the potassium intake is larger and is found in citrus fruit and chocolate. Potassium is absorbed throughout the small intestine; in the colon it is secreted in exchange for sodium ions. This serves two purposes; first to preserve sodium ions, and second to act as a minor excretory pathway in conditions of potassium excess.

Distribution

The potassium content of the body is about 50 mmol/kg, 95% of which is exchangeable. Most of the extracellular potassium is in bone (Table 2.2) and thus plasma levels are a poor index of overall potassium status. The total body content of potassium is mainly intracellular and is therefore related to body weight and provides a good indication of cellular mass. The total body potassium can be measured but this is rarely necessary in clinical practice.

Table 2.2 Approximate distribution of body potassium (% of whole)

Intracellular	90
Bone and connective tissue	8
Transcellular and interstitial	1.5
Plasma	0.5

Regulation and excretion

Despite widely differing intakes, the body content of potassium remains relatively constant in health. Control mechanisms are important because deficiency or excess can be lethal. Potassium is lost in

* this refers to the ECF as a percentage of body weight in infants, and in adults would be 0.2.

the gut, in sweat and from the kidney. The sweat potassium level is about 20 mmol/l and is higher in cystic fibrosis and hyperaldosteronism, but sweat losses are never of clinical significance. The renal regulation of potassium is most important. It is filtered at the glomerulus and is almost totally reabsorbed in the proximal tubule, only to be secreted again in the distal tubule. Most of the urinary potassium results from secretion rather than filtration, and in health the output balances the intake. The mechanisms that control the renal handling of potassium are less well understood than those for sodium. Potassium and hydrogen ions compete for exchange with urinary sodium under the influence of such factors as urine volume and flow, intracellular pH (which regulates intracellular potassium concentration) and secretion of aldosterone, which tends to conserve sodium at the expense of potassium.

Pathological states

Potassium deficiency may produce muscle weakness, cardiac arrhythmia and sudden death (Table 2.3). It usually results from excessive loss in vomiting, gastric aspiration or diarrhoea, or from

Table 2.3. Effects of extreme serum levels of potassium

Hypokalaemia	Hyperkalaemia
Plasma K^+ <3.0 mmol/l	Plasma K^+ >7.0 mmol/l
Muscle weakness	Virtually no specific symptoms
Paralytic ileus	Palpitations
Confusion	ECG changes:
Polyuria	
ECG changes:	

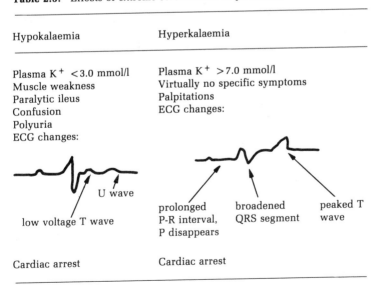

low voltage T wave — U wave

prolonged P-R interval, P disappears | broadened QRS segment | peaked T wave

| Cardiac arrest | Cardiac arrest |

diuretic therapy. Rarer causes are renal tubular diseases and Cushing's syndrome. Chronic potassium deficiency may cause renal tubular damage, interfering with renal concentrating capacity leading to alkalosis and resulting in continued potassium wastage. Hyperkalaemia usually results from poor excretion in renal failure, but other causes include increased tissue breakdown (such as during induction therapy in acute leukaemia) and congenital adrenal hyperplasia (21-hydroxylase deficiency).

As would be expected, the handling of potassium in disease is closely related to sodium and hydrogen ion concentration. When sodium is deficient it will be conserved at the expense of potassium; the urine will contain negligible sodium and appreciable potassium. In sodium excess there will be increased delivery of sodium to the distal tubule to be exchanged for potassium; the urine will contain appreciable sodium and potassium. With a systemic alkalosis such as caused by pyloric stenosis, potassium and H^+ are exchanged for sodium in the distal tubule, resulting in potassium loss even in the face of depletion of body potassium. Conversely, in an acidosis hydrogen ions are easily secreted and potassium tends to be retained even if there is hyperkalaemia.

Plasma potassium concentration

This represents only about 0.5% of the total body potassium and is not a good index of overall potassium balance. Variations in the plasma level are minimal compared with the intracellular pool, which cannot be measured by clinical techniques. As a working rule if the serum potassium is low then there is usually an overall deficit; however normal or high plasma levels may be observed when the total body potassium is low, for instance in uncontrolled diabetes with dehydration.

Chloride

Intake

Dietary chloride is ingested with sodium and is absorbed in the gut across an electrochemical gradient. Chloride has long been regarded as a passive ion, but there is now evidence of active chloride transport in the ascending limb of the loop of Henle (with sodium following passively) which may be blocked by diuretics such as frusemide and bumetanide.

Distribution

Chloride is an extracellular ion and very little is to be found in cells. The body content of chloride is 33 mmol/kg, distributed as shown in Table 2.4. Chloride and bicarbonate comprise 80% of the ECF anions and there is a reciprocal relationship between their concentrations.

Table 2.4 Approximate distribution of body chloride (% of whole)

Plasma and lymph	51
Bone and connective tissue	32
Intracellular } Transcellular }	16

Regulation and excretion

Some chloride is excreted in the gut and sweat, but it is mainly removed by the kidney. It tends to follow the pattern of sodium excretion and regulation (with the exception of the loop of Henle).

Pathological states

Chloride may be lost from the upper or lower gut; this usually occurs with sodium loss as in hypotonic dehydration, cystic fibrosis or pyloric stenosis. Sometimes it is lost in greater amounts than sodium or potassium with serious implications for treatment. When chloride is deficient in the glomerular filtrate proximal tubular reabsorption of sodium is inhibited, and the excess is presented for exchange with potassium and hydrogen ions in the distal tubule, resulting in hypokalaemia and alkalosis. In acidotic states chloride may be excreted separately from (and in greater amounts than) sodium, accompanied by hydrogen and ammonium ions. Diuretic drugs cause hypochloraemia; hyperchloraemia is seen with hypernatraemia and may complicate metabolic acidosis and ureteric reimplantation in the colon due to excessive absorption.

Plasma chloride concentration

This is helpful in calculating the anion gap (see p.5) and therefore the concentration of unmeasured ions. On its own the plasma chloride is of little significance as correction of abnormalities is passive, usually following restoration of acid/base balance and sodium homeostasis. Some laboratories do not measure it routinely.

Calcium

Detailed consideration of this ion is beyond the scope of this book, but a short discussion is required because of its relationship with other ions.

Intake

Milk is the principal dietary source of calcium. Active absorption takes place in the gut under the influence of vitamin D and parathyroid hormone and it can be blocked by substances which form insoluble salts of calcium, such as phosphate, oxalate and alkali.

Distribution

Calcium comprises about 1% of body weight, and about 99% of it is in bone where active turnover (remodelling and resorption) occurs at a rate of 100% per year in infancy. Approximately 50% of the calcium in the blood is protein-bound, but it is the unbound ionized form that is involved in processes such as blood coagulation, and muscle and nerve functions. The plasma concentration of calcium is regulated by the interactions of parathyroid hormone, vitamin D and calcium acting at different sites (Table 2.5).

Regulation and excretion

Glomerular filtrate contains free calcium ions and reabsorption occurs along the length of the nephrons — but mainly in the proximal tubule and loop of Henle — by a similar transport mechanism to sodium. An independent system in the distal nephron exerts a major influence on the final calcium content of urine. An increase in ECF volume and the use of diuretics such as frusemide promote calciuria.

Table 2.5 The effects of hormones on various tissues and the consequent effects on plasma calcium levels

Hormone/vitamin	Concentration in blood	Site of action	Effect on plasma calcium levels
Calcitonin	raised lowered	Bone	lowered raised
Vitamin D	raised lowered	Gut	raised lowered
Parathyroid hormone (and Vitamin D)	raised lowered	Kidney	raised lowered

Pathological states

Hypercalcaemia is rarely caused by a primary derangement of body fluids or electrolyte balance, but hypercalcaemia, by interfering with renal concentrating powers, may cause a massive diuresis and dehydration. Hypertonic hypernatraemic dehydration is often accompanied by hypocalcaemia which may cause the convulsions that sometimes complicate this condition; the mechanism is unknown.

~ 50% is protein bound.

Plasma calcium concentration

This is maintained within a small range and the level measured in the routine laboratory is the total, bound and unbound. Since it is the ionized fraction which is physiologically important it would be helpful to have this measured, but it is technically more difficult. The total plasma calcium level is influenced by the level of plasma proteins and when these are deficient, as in liver disease or the nephrotic syndrome, the plasma calcium will be low. Conversely, elevation of plasma proteins causes a rise in plasma calcium, as may occur due to venous stasis when the arm is squeezed for venepuncture. The level of ionized calcium is altered by pH changes: acidosis increases ionization and alkalosis decreases it. This explains why tetany may occur during excessively rapid correction of acidosis with alkali.

Phosphate

Intake

Phosphorus is widely distributed throughout all foodstuffs, particularly meat and milk, and an average western diet contains sufficient for health. It is absorbed in the small intestine; the presence of excessive calcium interferes with its absorption and vice versa. Neonatal hypocalcaemic tetany was common when babies were fed on full and half cream milks with a high phosphate content.

Distribution

Most of the plasma phosphate is unbound and exists mainly as the divalent anion HPO_4^{2-}, with about 20% as the monovalent $H_2PO_4^-$ anion. It is the most important urinary buffer in the regulation of hydrogen ion concentration (see Chapter 3). The ECF content is small; most phosphate (75%) is sequestered in bone and the rest is intracellular, mainly in muscle, providing the source of phosphorus for ATP formation. The total body content of phosphate is about 20 g in the full term baby compared with 650 g in the adult.

Regulation and excretion

Phosphate metabolism is subject to a number of different controls. Its absorption is influenced by circulating vitamin D and its plasma level is regulated by vitamin D, the direct action of calcitonin and indirectly by the phosphaturic action of parathyroid hormone. Phosphate handling by the kidney has some similarities with sodium and glucose: since it is mainly unbound, phosphate is filtered at the glomerulus and 90% is reabsorbed, principally in the proximal tubule. Factors promoting sodium excretion, such as diuretics and expansion of the ECF, also cause phosphaturia. Glycosuria reduces the tubular ability to reabsorb phosphate. Other hormones involved in phosphate excretion are growth hormone and sex hormones such as testosterone.

Pathological states

Hyperphosphataemia

As phosphate excretion is heavily dependent on the glomerular filtration rate (GFR) plasma levels rise in renal insufficiency. This probably happens early in the condition but clinical effects do not occur until the GFR is below about 30 ml/min/1.73m². Aluminium and calcium bind phosphorus in the gut, and compounds such as aluminium hydroxide and calcium carbonate are given to patients with chronic renal failure and hyperphosphataemia. This restricts intestinal absorption, and thus lowers the plasma level and prevents metastatic calcification. Hyperphosphataemia is also a feature of hypoparathyroidism resulting from deficiency of phosphaturic parathyroid hormone.

Hypophosphataemia

The most common cause is administration of phosphorus-free fluids for more than a few days. It is also a feature of diabetes mellitus with heavy glycosuria. Patients receiving prolonged intravenous fluid therapy need phosphate supplements. Diseases causing hypophosphataemia are hyperparathyroidism and vitamin D-resistant (phosphaturic) rickets.

Plasma phosphate concentration

The phosphorus level is age dependent (Table 2.6) and care is required in the interpretation of laboratory results, particularly when the reference ranges are those given for adults. There is a diurnal variation and the level is highest just after a meal.

Table 2.6 Mean plasma phosphate (mmol/l)

Birth	1.90	12 months	1.55
7 days	2.55	5 years	1.37
6 months	1.67	Adult	1.22

Magnesium

Intake

As magnesium is an important cation in enzymatic function it would be anticipated that the greatest requirements occur at times of growth. About 30% of the intake is absorbed and about 10 mmol is required daily for growth. Cereals and vegetables are notable sources of magnesium but losses may occur during processing.

Distribution

This is mainly in bone and muscle cells (Table 2.7). The infant contains about 10 mmol/kg body weight and the adult about 15 mmol/kg.

Table 2.7   Approximate distribution of body magnesium (% of whole)

Bone	60
Intracellular	39
Extracellular	1

Regulation and excretion

The kidney provides the most important control of magnesium levels, and the ion is handled similarly to calcium and sodium with about 60% of plasma magnesium being unbound to protein and available for filtration. About 30% of the intake is excreted but this may be modified by drugs and diet. Parathyroid hormone increases the plasma level of magnesium (as well as calcium) by promoting tubular reabsoption and mobilization from ICF and bone.

Pathological states

Hypermagnesaemia causes neurological and respiratory depression and cardiotoxicity, and usually results from acute renal failure or excessive therapeutic administration. It is treated by promoting a diuresis and the careful administration of calcium salts. Low levels of magnesium occur in severe malnutrition, either primary malnutrition or as a consequence of disease, malabsorption or alcoholism in adults. Hypomagnesaemia in the newborn is usually associated with maternal diabetes, cow's milk feeds, and following exchange transfusion. It causes a clinical picture similar to

hypocalcaemia (which may accompany it) with neuromuscular irritability sometimes progressing to convulsions. Treatment is by
giving magnesium salts.

Plasma magnesium concentration

As with potassium, plasma magnesium levels are a poor guide to
body stores as such a small proportion is in the ECF. No correction
for plasma protein level or venous stasis is required. The mean level
is 0.87 mmol/l at birth, falling to 0.83 mmol/l at 10 years old.

3

Acid/Base Balance

Just as the body fluid and electrolyte concentrations are constantly changing under the influence of many different controls, so is the hydrogen ion (H^+) concentration. Regulation of this ion in the ECF is particularly important because the ICF H^+ concentration is dependent on it, and because the various and vital intracellular functions are very sensitive to changes in H^+ concentrations.

Terminology

The pH notation has been traditionally used to express hydrogen ion concentration because it is present in the body in much smaller amounts than other ions (Table 3.1). pH is the negative logarithm of H^+ concentration, i.e. H^+ concentration = 40 nanomol/l or 4×10^{-8}, $\therefore$ pH = $-\log (4 \times 10^{-8})$

$$= -(\log 4 + \log 10^{-8})$$
$$= -\log 4 - \log 10^{-8}$$
$$= -(0.6) - (-8)$$
$$= -0.6 + 8$$
$$= 7.4$$

Table 3.2 shows the relationship between H^+ and pH. It can be seen

Table 3.1 Various ionic concentrations

Ion	Plasma concentration (mmol/l)
Na^+	140
K^+	4.5
H^+	0.00004 (40 nmol/l)

Table 3.2 To show the relationship between H^+ and pH

H^+ (nmol/l)	pH
20	7.70
40	7.40
50	7.30
60	7.22
70	7.16
80	7.10
100	7.00
120	6.92

24

that if the H^+ value is doubled or halved the pH changes by 0.3 units. If the pH is changed by 1 unit (a very unlikely clinical event) then the H^+ concentration changes tenfold. In future acid/base balance may be expressed clinically as H^+; the pH notation is still widely accepted and will be employed in this book. The normal pH of ECF is 7.4 ± 0.03 and of the ICF about 7.1. These values are altered by disease, and the term acid/base balance is used to indicate the result of controlling mechanisms.

Acids, bases and buffers

The amount of free hydrogen ion is very small; however the amount of ionizable hydrogen ion is much greater and is mainly present in association with anions or uncharged compounds, some of which are shown in Table 3.3. Those substances which donate H^+ in solution are called acids; those that readily give up H^+ are strong acids, for example hydrochloric acid; and those that only dissociate to a small extent are weak acids — carbonic acid. Compounds that accept H^+ are known as bases. These relationships are shown in Figure 3.1. A buffer is a system that can bind or release H^+ in solution, thereby maintaining the pH of the solution constant despite the addition of acid or base.

Table 3.3 Blood buffering agents

HHB	(haemoglobin)
HProt	(protein)
H_2CO_3	(carbonic acid)
H_3PO_4	(phosphate)

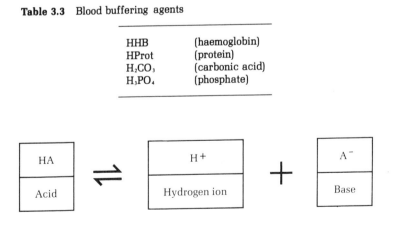

Figure 3.1 The relationship between acid, H^+ and base.

The system shown in Figure 3.1 should be considered further:

$$HA \rightleftharpoons H^+ + A^-$$

when acid is added

$$HA \leftarrow H^+ \overset{\diagup\ H^+}{+ A^-}$$

the excess H^+ will combine with base A^- and the equation shifts to the left, thus damping down the potential rise in H^+ concentration or fall in pH.

The law of mass action states that the product of the concentrations of the products (H^+ and A^-) in a chemical reaction divided by the product of the concentration of the reactants at equilibrium (HA) is a constant, K, where:

$$K = \frac{(H^+)(A^-)}{HA}$$

Thus if a large amount of H^+ is added to the system the concentration of the base A^- must decrease and the concentration of HA increase to keep the ratio constant. From this equation can be derived the Henderson–Hasselbalch equation:

$$pH = K + \log \frac{(A^-)}{HA}$$

If the bicarbonate/carbonic acid buffer system is used as an example:

$$\frac{(H^+)(HCO_3^-)}{H_2CO_3} = K$$

and H_2CO_3 is in equilibrium with dissolved carbon dioxide as $H_2O + CO_2 \rightleftharpoons H_2CO_3$; this reaction is catalyzed by the enzyme carbonic anhydrase. It can be seen that the addition of H^+ to the system will result in a decrease in HCO_3^- — a base deficit — and a corresponding rise in manufactured H_2CO_3. The H_2CO_3 will then dissociate to CO_2 and H_2O, and the partial pressure (or concentration) of CO_2 in the blood would rise were it not for compensatory hyperventilation which blows off the CO_2, and the P_{CO_2} will therefore stabilize. During this time there will be a transient fall in pH (or rise in H^+ concentration) until the compensatory process is complete. Using the Henderson–Hasselbalch equation:

$$pH = pK + \log \frac{(bicarbonate)}{carbonic\ acid}$$

but as carbonic acid is in equilibrium with dissolved carbon dioxide, which varies with the partial pressure of carbon dioxide (P_{CO_2}), the concentration of P_{CO_2} can be substituted as:

$$pH = pK + \log \frac{HCO_3^-}{P_{CO_2}} \quad \text{or} \quad pH \, \alpha \, \frac{HCO_3}{P_{CO_2}}$$

Other important buffers in the blood are the plasma proteins and haemoglobin and in the urine, phosphate, ammonium ion and bicarbonate systems.

Control of acid/base balance

Dietary protein is the principal source of H^+, the remainder is derived from incomplete metabolism of fat and carbohydrate (when the latter compounds are completely metabolized they form H_2O and CO_2). Approximately 70 mmol of H^+ is excreted in the urine per day.

There are two major controls regulating the acid/base balance system; the quick-reacting buffer systems, and slower-reacting compensatory and corrective changes in lungs and kidneys which allow excretion of H^+ and regeneration of buffer.

Lung

The lungs directly influence the bicarbonate buffer system only, although other systems are affected by consequent changes in H^+ concentration. The reaction in respiratory control is: $CO_2 + H_2O \leftrightharpoons H_2CO_3 \leftrightharpoons H^+ + HCO_3^-$, and the partial pressure of CO_2 in the alveolus is directly related to the concentration of CO_2 in the blood (P_{CO_2}). The lung has two methods of control: increased and decreased ventilation. Increased ventilation will reduce the P_{CO_2} and the H^+, thus elevating the pH: $\downarrow CO_2 + H_2O \leftarrow H_2CO_3 \leftarrow \downarrow H^+ + HCO_3^-$

Conversely, decreased ventilation will cause the reaction to shift to the right, increasing H^+ and lowering the pH: $\uparrow CO_2 + H_2O \rightarrow H_2CO_3 \rightarrow \uparrow H^+ + HCO_3^-$

Kidney

As has been seen the blood buffers and lung provide a temporary means of coping with an acid load and maintaining homeostasis. However surplus H^+ must be excreted and bicarbonate regenerated. These functions are carried out in the kidney. H^+ is secreted by the proximal and distal tubular cells and thus makes the urine acid. H^+ transport is an active process and electroneutrality is maintained by sodium reabsorption. The lowest urinary pH that can be achieved in man is about 4.5. If there were no other method for excreting H^+ then this pH would be achieved and no further acid excretion could occur. There are three other urinary buffer systems by which further acid excretion is achieved.

Bicarbonate system

Most of the secreted H^+ reacts with filtered bicarbonate in the proximal tubule to form carbonic acid and thence CO_2 and H_2O (Figure 3.2). The CO_2 is absorbed into the tubular cell when it combines with water under the influence of carbonic anhydrase, generating bicarbonate which diffuses back into the blood. Thus H^+ is secreted and HCO_3^- reabsorbed.

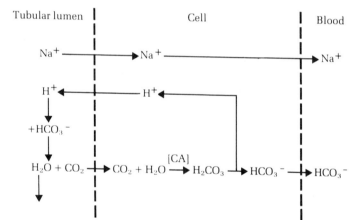

Figure 3.2 The bicarbonate buffer system of the proximal renal tubule. CA = carbonic anhydrase.

Phosphate system

This is less important than the bicarbonate system in the proximal tubule as the concentration of phosphate is very much lower. In the distal tubule the phosphate concentration is higher and the reactions shown in Figure 3.3 occur, generating phosphate for excretion and bicarbonate to be reabsorbed into the blood. The amount of H^+ that reacts with non-bicarbonate buffer constitutes the titrable acidity of the urine; it will be appreciated that this is only a minute amount of the total acid secreted.

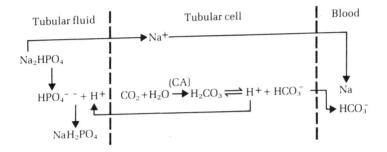

Figure 3.3 The phosphate buffer system of the proximal renal tubule. CA = carbonic anhydrase.

Ammonia system

In states of increased H^+ concentration the distal tubular cell metabolizes glutamine to form ammonia. The ammonia diffuses into the tubular lumen and buffers H^+ (Figure 3.4) to form NH_4^+ which is unable to diffuse back into the tubular cell.

Intracellular acid/base control

The cell wall is less permeable to anions such as bicarbonate than to unchanged molecules such as H_2CO_3 (and therefore CO_2). Cations are exchanged by active transport. Therefore pulmonary changes of the P_{CO_2} will affect cell pH rapidly, but changes in intracellular H^+ concentration will be slower if acid is added to the ECF and allowed to diffuse.

Pathological states

Four basic abnormalities of acid/base balance are recognized: metabolic (non-respiratory) acidosis and alkalosis occur when there is a primary increase or decrease in H^+ production in the body or a

Chapter 3

primary decrease or increase in HCO_3^- or other buffers. Respiratory acidosis and alkalosis occur following changes in respiration resulting in an increase or decrease in the P_{CO_2}. Table 3.4 summarizes these changes.

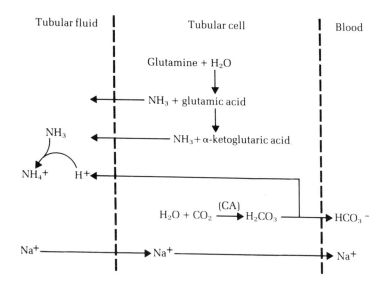

Figure 3.4 The renal ammonium buffer system. CA = carbonic anhydrase.

Metabolic acidosis

One major cause is from increased production or deficient excretion of H^+, when the presence of anions such as sulphate and ß-OH butyrate will cause an increase in the anion gap (see p.5). The other principle cause results from an excessive loss of bicarbonate, such as occurs in severe diarrhoea and proximal renal tubular acidosis. The additional H^+ is buffered by the bicarbonate system forming H_2CO_3, and hence CO_2, which is excreted through the lungs, and H_2O. Renal compensation occurs through ammonium formation and H^+ excretion, and bicarbonate is regenerated.

The clinical effect is of deep sighing breathing (Kussmaul respiration) such as is seen in diabetic ketoacidosis. Treatment is of the primary cause, such as with insulin and fluid in diabetes. Reversal

Table 3.4 Pathological changes in acid/base status

	Clinical condition	Acid/base changes		Clinical symptoms or signs
		Primary	Compensatory	
Metabolic acidosis	Diabetes mellitus	↓pH (↑H^+) ↓HCO_3^-	↓P_{CO_2}	Increased respiration
Metabolic alkalosis	Pyloric stenosis	↑pH (↓H^+) ↑HCO_3^-	↑P_{CO_2}	Decreased respiration
Respiratory acidosis	Terminal status asthmaticus	↓pH (↑H^+) ↑P_{CO_2}	↑HCO_3^-	Drowsiness
Respiratory alkalosis	Hysterical overbreathing	↑pH (↓H^+) ↓P_{CO_2}	↓HCO_3^-	Tetany

of the acidosis may be aided by administration of sodium bicarbonate. This is not entirely safe because of the sodium content which causes an increased osmolality of the ECF, stimulating a rapid shift of water from the ICF.

The clinical criteria for use are controversial but with a pH of less than 7.10, with circulatory failure or undesirably slow response to therapy of the primary condition then sodium bicarbonate can be given according to the formula: 0.3 × body weight × base deficit, or 0.3 × body weight × (15 − plasma bicarbonate). 0.3 represents the ECF volume into which the bicarbonate must diffuse; it varies with age (see Table 1.2). (15 − plasma bicarbonate) allows for correction up to a plasma bicarbonate of 15 mmol/l; other compensatory mechanisms will perform the final correction. In diabetic ketoacidosis bicarbonate administration may contribute to the profound fall in the plasma potassium which will occur due to the administration of insulin and water.

Metabolic alkalosis

In metabolic alkalosis there is excessive loss of H^+, as in pyloric stenosis, or excessive influx of bicarbonate exogenously by ingestion or infusion. The plasma bicarbonate and pH rise; there may be a compensatory fall in ventilation allowing a small rise in P_{CO_2}. Plasma levels of potassium and chloride are low, and in severe pyloric stenosis causing sodium and potassium depletion the renal tubule will secrete potassium and H^+ in exchange for sodium, causing a paradoxical aciduria in the presence of a systemic alkalosis. Symptoms are usually of weakness, cramps and perhaps tetany from a reduced level of ionized calcium. Specific treatment of the alkalosis is rarely required after restoration of depleted water, sodium and potassium. Rarely, a persisting low chloride may require treatment with ammonium or calcium chloride.

Respiratory acidosis

If insufficient carbon dioxide is excreted from the lungs the P_{CO_2} will rise and cause an increase in H^+ concentration and acidosis. Compensation occurs by increased renal ammonia and H^+ secretion, thereby generating extra bicarbonate to counter the increased P_{CO_2} and to restore the pH toward normal. Respiratory acidosis is seen in poisoning by CNS depressants or respiratory failure from pneumonia, or advanced status asthmaticus. The main symptom of a high P_{CO_2} is headache from cerebral vasodilatation and a hyperdynamic circulation. There is no specific treatment other than for the primary cause of respiratory depression and CO_2 retention.

Respiratory alkalosis

Overbreathing may be induced deliberately, such as by increasing mechanically-assisted ventilation in cases of cerebral oedema; it may occur with hysteria or by the direct effects of salicylate on the respiratory centre. The effect is to wash out CO_2 from the lungs, thereby lowering the P_{CO_2} and H^+, and raising the pH. To compensate, H^+ released from intracellular buffers combines with bicarbonate whilst renal bicarbonate excretion increases. The symptoms in respiratory alkalosis are usually those of the primary condition but a low P_{CO_2} does induce paraesthesia. Treatment is of the cause of hyperventilation.

Mixed disturbances

Sometimes there is more than one cause for deranged acid/base states, for example metabolic and respiratory acidosis may coexist in the respiratory distress syndrome of infancy. The drop in pH is greater than in a single disturbance because the compensatory

Table 3.5 Mixed acid/base disorders

Disorder	Clinical condition	pH
Metabolic acidosis Respiratory acidosis	Respiratory distress syndrome	Profoundly reduced
Metabolic acidosis Respiratory alkalosis	Salicylate poisoning	High, normal or low
Metabolic alkalosis Respiratory acidosis	Diuretic therapy in cor pulmonale	High, normal or low
Metabolic alkalosis Respiratory alkalosis	Unlikely to occur in a single condition in children	Greatly raised

mechanisms (decreasing P_{CO_2} in metabolic acidosis or increasing bicarbonate in respiratory acidosis) cannot act or may worsen the acid/base status. Other examples are seen in Table 3.5.

Assessment of acid/base balance

This should preferably be done using an air-free syringe to collect arterial blood which is sent to the laboratory on ice; arterialized capillary samples can be used. The results obtained are the pH, P_{CO_2} and P_{O_2}, from which the standard bicarbonate and base excess or deficit are calculated. The standard bicarbonate is the concentration of bicarbonate at a temperature of 37°C and a P_{CO_2} of 40 mmHg (c. 5320 Pa) — that is an assessment of the metabolic component alone. The base excess or deficit, positive in alkalosis and negative in acidosis, is the amount of acid or base required to restore 1 litre of blood to normal acid/base status at a P_{CO_2} of 40 mmHg, and is a measure of metabolic disturbance.

Interpretation of theoretical acid/base data — examples

DATA	INTERPRETATION
1 pH 7.0 HCO₃ 4 mmol/l P_{CO_2} 25 mmHg Base deficit 12 mmol	acidosis low HCO₃, low P_{CO_2}, considerable base deficit. ∴ metabolic acidosis. Consider treatment with bicarbonate according to formula: base deficit or (15 − plasma bicarbonate) × 0.3 × body weight.
2 pH 7.52 HCO₃ 35 P_{CO_2} 45 Base excess 10	alkalosis high bicarbonate, modestly raised P_{CO_2}, base excess. ∴ metabolic alkalosis should improve with correction of water and electrolyte balance.
3 pH 7.20 HCO₃ 30 P_{CO_2} 75 Base excess − 4	acidosis high bicarbonate, high P_{CO_2}, modest base deficit. ∴ respiratory acidosis; treat by improving ventilation.

4 pH 7.50
   HCO₃ 23
   Pco₂ 25
   Base excess + 1

} alkalosis
  normal bicarbonate, low P_{CO_2}, little change in base excess. Respiratory alkalosis: will improve spontaneously unless caused by automatic ventilation of lungs.

5 pH 7.0
   HCO₃ 9
   Pco₂ 80
   Base deficit − 8

} acidosis
  low bicarbonate and negative base excess indicate metabolic acidosis. Very high P_{CO_2} indicates respiratory acidosis. This is a mixed acidosis (respiratory and metabolic).

6 pH 7.27
   HCO₂ 9
   Pco₂ 17
   Base excess − 6

} acidosis
  moderately low bicarbonate and negative base excess but grossly low P_{CO_2}. Mixed respiratory alkalosis and metabolic acidosis; latter predominating, e.g. salicylate intoxication.

4

Water and Electrolyte Requirements

The following description applies to children outside the neonatal period. Fluid therapy in the newborn child is considered in Chapter 13.

Routes of fluid administration

Oral or nasogastric tube

This is the preferred method of fluid and electrolyte administration in mild gastroenteritis and dehydration. If the child is vomiting, or fluid loss continues to be greater than can be supplied by mouth, then an alternative technique is required.

Intravenous

In the UK this is the most widely used route of access to the circulation. Scalp, hand or foot veins are used in infants, and arm veins in older children. The advantages of intravenous administration are that the therapy is given directly into the circulation — particularly important where there is circulatory failure — and that fluid and drugs can be given in precise amounts and rates. The drawbacks are that venous cannulation can be difficult with a plump or collapsed infant, infection from the cannula may cause local phlebitis or disseminated infection, and the head shaving required for scalp vein cannulation may be distressing to the parents.

Rectal infusions (proctoclysis)

Introduced by an Irish surgeon (J. B. Murphy) in 1906, this technique has largely been abandoned. In cases such as pyloric stenosis with vomiting where the lower bowel is normal, it is an easy method for providing maintenance fluids pre-operatively.

Subcutaneous infusion (hypodermaclysis)

With this method there is poor absorption if there is circulatory failure, and it is now rarely used in the UK. Suitable sites are the subscapular region, axillae and lower abdominal wall.

Intraperitoneal

In difficult circumstances where intravenous cannulation is impossible this route can be used, although absorption may be erratic with a compromised circulation. It used to be a popular method of giving blood transfusions.

Water and electrolyte requirements

Children exist in a state of balance; dietary intake of water, electrolytes and nutrition is balanced by the demands of metabolism, growth, elimination and excretion. In health these demands are met by the consumption of normal amounts of food and drink and little thought is given to the balance unless some disorder such as anorexia nervosa or obesity occurs. In disease dietary intake may not be taken or absorbed and water, electrolytes and nutrition must therefore be given by some other means. These are called *maintenance requirements*; unconscious patients who have no other complications need their maintenance requirements calculated and administered, usually via a nasogastric tube.

If there is excessive loss of water, as in diabetic ketoacidosis, or electrolyte, such as in pyloric stenosis, then this deficit must first be replaced. Continuing loss, as in an enteric fistula, must not be allowed to become a deficit, but must be anticipated and supplied in addition to the maintenance fluid. The sum of these is the *total requirement*. In health the maintenance requirement is the same as the total requirement. These relationships are shown in Figure 4.1.

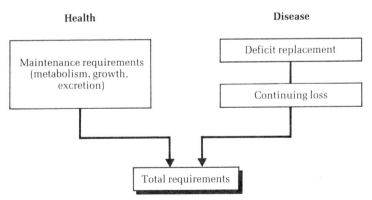

Figure 4.1 Nutritional (fluid, electrolyte and energy) requirements.

Maintenance water

Volume

Water is taken in through the diet, is consumed during metabolism, is produced endogenously from oxidation, and is eliminated and excreted in the stools and urine and from the skin and lungs. Older children and adults will regulate their water intake depending on their thirst, which is a manifestation of the total body water volume and solute concentration (osmolality), and involves the normal relationship of the hypothalamus and cerebral cortex with osmoreceptors. These controls can be overriden such as in emotional disorders of compulsive water drinking. Unconscious or profoundly handicapped patients will not be able to regulate water balance automatically and their requirements must be calculated. Chronic underhydration and hypernatraemia is sometimes seen in such patients — it is not usually due to a urinary-concentrating deficit, but more often to a deficit in water administration.

Influence of body size

It is obvious that water requirements of a newborn baby and an adult will be very different; if the water requirement for an adult is given to a baby then it will develop fluid-overload, heart failure and pulmonary oedema. Some measure is required to scale down the requirements; an age relationship might be considered but this does not allow for the great differences of body build with age. The most precise estimates are those based on total energy expenditure in health or disease. This is not easy to calculate in everyday clinical practice and so, accepting some error, fluid balance is related to surface area, using a height/weight nomogram, or to weight and age (Table 4.1). This may give a higher requirement than the metabolic rate method, especially of water intake in older children. The minimum daily requirement of water is equivalent to that lost from the skin and lungs, and in the urine and stools.

Renal water loss

The *obligatory urine volume* is that amount of water required to excrete the waste products of metabolism without the body fluids becoming excessively concentrated. This depends on the amount of waste solute and the capacity of the kidneys to concentrate urine.

Table 4.1   Maintenance water requirements (in ml/kg BW/24 hours)

Age (years)	Water
0-0.5	150
0.5-3	100
3-6	90
7-12	70
Over 12	50

The *solute load* is mainly composed of nitrogenous compounds (urea) and electrolytes; the basal urea contribution to urine concentration is about 4 mmol/420 kJ (100 kcal) expended, and the electrolyte contribution (sodium, potassium and chloride) about 10 mmol/420 kJ, giving a total renal solute load of about 15 mmol/420 kJ. This can be excreted in about 10 ml water/420 kJ at maximum urine concentration, but a basal rate of 55 ml water/420 kJ will allow a urine concentration of 200-300 mmol/kg and avoid excessive renal concentration or dilution. When related to weight rather than energy expended this volume varies from about 50 ml/kg in a six-month baby to 25 ml/kg in adolescents. In hypercatabolic states or conditions of excessive dietary intake the solute load and solvent (water) requirement will be several times greater.

Renal concentrating capacity varies with age and usual intake. A breast fed infant will have a low solute load and will only be required to maximally concentrate the urine to 600 mmol/kg, whereas a baby fed with cow's milk and with a greater solute load will have the capacity to concentrate urine to over 1000 mmol/kg. The capacity of the kidney to clear solute is expressed as the osmolal clearance and is:

$$C_{osm} = \frac{U_{osm} \times V}{P_{osm}}$$

where U_{osm} = osmolality of urine, V = urine volume in unit time, and P_{osm} = plasma osmolality.

If the urine volume is limited because of excessive loss elsewhere (e.g. diarrhoea) the concentration of solute and electrolytes in the blood will rise when the U_{osm} has reached its ceiling. In conditions such as diabetes insipidus where the limit of U_{osm} is much lower, a correspondingly greater water intake is required.

Insensible water loss (IWL)

This is the evaporative loss of water from the skin and lungs. In infancy it consumes almost 50% of the water requirement, but this proportion declines with age to about 25% in the adult. The IWL contributes to heat loss — about 25% body heat being lost by this route. The conversion of 1 ml water to vapour requires 2.45 kJ (0.58 kcal), and about 4 ml water are evaporated for every 42 kJ (10 kcal) metabolized. At rest more water is lost from the skin than the lungs but this will change in conditions such as hyperventilation in salicylate poisoning. At an environmental humidity of 100%, IWL from the lungs will cease, water and heat cannot be lost and the body temperature may rise and fluid requirements will fall. If nebulizers are used for a long period there is a risk of excessive pulmonary absorption of water and haemodilution.

The IWL will vary with the metabolic rate and where this is increased, particularly in feverish illness, heat production and IWL will be greater. A rise in body temperature of 1°C will increase the metabolic rate and IWL by 10%; thus for every 1° above 37°C 10 ml/kg additional water is required. Conditions causing coma, sedatives and hypothyroidism will decrease the metabolic rate and IWL.

The allowance for IWL will, like the renal water allowance, vary with size: maintenance IWL requirements for a six-month baby will be 40 ml/kg and at adolescence 20 ml/kg.

Gastrointestinal water loss

Although 85% of faeces is water, the total daily loss from this route is small in health. Infants lose about 5 ml/kg/24 hours and adolescents 2.5 ml/kg/24 hours. During episodes of diarrhoea greater volumes are lost — up to 30 ml/kg/24 hours; vomiting, enteric fistulae and nasogastric suction will also result in excessive water loss.

Summary

The water allowance for obligatory urine volume, IWL, stool water and growth is termed the minimal water requirement; this would balance a minimal water intake, assuming maximal powers of renal concentration. Intake is obviously greater to allow a margin of safety in renal water concentration. These relationships are summarized in Figure 4.2. See Table 4.1. for suggested maintenance water volumes for age and weight.

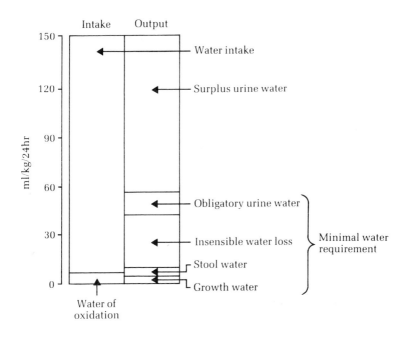

Figure 4.2 Water balance in infancy, measured in ml/kg/24 hours.

Maintenance fluid composition

Most electrolyte loss takes place through the kidneys, and with normal renal function there is a great variation in electrolyte excretion. Recommendations for maintenance are largely based upon the electrolyte content of normal dietary constituents, for example breast milk. In health small amounts of electrolyte are lost in stool and sweat, but pathological conditions such as diarrhoea or cystic fibrosis will increase these. There is negligible electrolyte loss in IWL. Sodium and potassium are replaced as the chloride salts; the excess of chloride is of no clinical importance. Calcium, magnesium and phosphorus are not required for short term maintenance therapy, but when protracted nutrition is required they must be included in amounts adequate for growth. Table 4.2 gives the maintenance electrolyte requirements.

Table 4.2 Maintenance electrolyte requirements (in mmol/kg BW/24 hours)

Age (years)	Na	K	Ca	Mg	P	Cl
0–0.5	2.5	2.5	1.5	1	1.5	2.5
0.5–3	2.5	2.5	1.5	1	1.5	2.5
3–6	2.0	2.0	1.5	1	1.5	2.0
7–12	1.5	1.5	1.5	1	1.5	1.5
Over 12	1.5	1.5	1.5	1	1.5	1.5

The concentration or osmolality of oral fluids can be varied but intravenous fluids should be isotonic with plasma; it is convenient to mix the electrolyte and basal energy requirements in water. A convenient oral solution is marketed as Dioralyte powder and its reconstituted composition shown in Table 4.3 (there are other similar commercial preparations — Dextrolyte, Electrosol, Rehydrat). A widely used maintenance parenteral solution is 0.18% NaCl and 4.3% dextrose whose composition is shown in Table 4.4. There may not be any potassium in this solution; when potassium is required it should be added to an appropriate concentration using an aseptic technique, and great care should be taken to ensure that the potassium is well mixed in the solution. Potassium should never be given undiluted because of the risk of cardiotoxicty, and the maximum desirable concentration is 30 mmol/l intravenous fluid. Ampoules of 1.5 g KCl in 20 ml supply 20 mmol of potassium and chloride respectively, to be dissolved in 500 ml fluid.

Table 4.3 Composition of 1 litre of Dioralyte*

Na$^+$	K$^+$	Cl$^-$	HCO$_3^-$	Glucose	Energy	Osmolality
35 mmol	20 mmol	37 mmol	18 mmol	222 mmol (40 g)	672 kJ (160 kcal)	310 mmol/kg

*Five sachets dissolved in 1 litre of boiled water.

Table 4.4 Composition of 1 litre of 0.18% NaCl and 4.3% dextrose

Na$^+$	K$^+$	Cl$^-$	HCO$_3^-$	Glucose	Energy	Osmolality
31 mmol	0 mmol	31 mmol	0 mmol	235 mmol (43 g)	722.4 kJ (172 kcal)	301 mmol/kg

Maintenance energy

It is unnecessary to supply full energy requirements for short periods of poor nutrition, such as in nonspecific gastroenteritis in the UK, as the average child will have adequate energy stores. Sufficient glucose should be given to prevent ketosis and to minimize catabolism of tissue protein; this will be supplied in the proprietary oral rehydration solutions. Glucose in oral solutions also promotes sodium absorption by the gut. If diarrhoea continues, or normal food is withheld for more than 3–5 days, then tissue catabolism will occur and enteral or parenteral nutrition will need to be considered. These are described in Chapter 11.

Rate of administration

Oral

The total daily requirement can be given at intervals to suit the child or its attendants. If vomiting is likely then small volumes should be given and flavoured with orange or blackcurrant. When the child's condition is stable milk may be offered.

Parenteral

Intravenous cannulae are likely to remain patent when fluid is flowing through — otherwise they should be filled with heparinized fluid. In the short term the total daily volume is divided by 24 and the result infused per hour. For longer term fluid therapy, 24 hour requirements can be infused over a shorter period, leaving the day or night free.

Monitoring

Certain observations should be made before starting therapy and at regular intervals during treatment. Suggested observations are:

1 Body weight — perhaps the most important. Ideally the same person should measure this using the same scales. The frequency will be dictated by the size of child and underlying conditions, but in most acute illnesses this should be done at least daily.

2 Clinical examination for the characteristic signs of over- and underhydration, including the blood pressure.

3 Meticulous review of intake and output charts for volumes, an approximate calculation of composition and a calculation of balance.

4 Measurement of plasma urea and electrolytes — once or twice during an acute self-limiting episode of diarrhoea but daily during acute oliguric renal failure. Other measurements such as liver function tests, calcium, phosphate, etc. will be required in longer term nutrition.

Modified maintenance requirements

In disease states there may be excessive fluid and electrolyte loss; at presentation the deficiency needs to be made up and if loss continues this must be added to the daily maintenance fluid requirement. Ideally the volume lost per unit time should be measured, and the fluid analysed for the electrolyte content and the equivalent replaced by mouth or intravenously.

In practice gastric aspirate and small intestinal drainage is replaced volume for volume by commercially available fluids as shown in Table 4.5. Although the figures given in the analyses of commercially available fluids do not entirely correspond to calculated electrolyte loss they are close enough for everyday use; providing renal function is normal the kidneys will do the fine regulation. Excessive stool loss may be compensated for by giving extra fluid volume, as shown in Table 4.5. Continuing urinary loss of water and electrolyte occurs following acute renal failure and after relief of urinary obstruction. Volume for volume replacement should be given and the urinary electrolytes measured and replaced. In hot weather children with cystic fibrosis have a high obligatory salt loss in sweat, and salt supplements should be given.

Sometimes the maintenance fluid must be reduced. Oliguric renal failure is an example, and the total fluid intake in such cir-

Table 4.5 Composition of replacement fluids

	Na (mmol/l)	K⁺ (mmol/l)	Cl (mmol/l)	HCO₃ (mmol/l)	Fluid composition
Gastric aspirate					
Theoretical requirement	20–80	5–20	100–150		
Practical solution	77	20	90		0.45% saline + 1.5 g (20 mmol) KCL/l
Small intestinal drainage					
Theoretical requirement	100–140	5–15	90–130	30	
Practical solution	77	20	90	30	0.45% saline + 1.5 g (20 mmol) KCL/l + 30 ml 8.4% NaHCO₃/l (or 50% strength Darrow's solution)
Lower gastrointestinal tract — diarrhoea					
Theoretical requirements	10–90	10–30	10–110		
Practical Solution	31	20	31		0.18% saline/4.3% dextrose + 1.5 g (20 mmol) KCL/l

cumstances is insensible loss plus urine output (plus any loss in gastric aspirate or diarrhoea). In infants under one year old IWL plus stool water (assuming no diarrhoea) is 40 ml/kg; in older children it equals 20 ml/kg. Potassium should be given with great caution in oliguric states.

5

Solving Water and Electrolyte Problems

In this chapter use is made of the physiological principles discussed in Chapters 1–4 to construct a general approach to water and electrolyte disorders. Figure 5.1 shows a scheme for their management and it is useful to use this framework until one is proficient at assessing fluid and electrolyte balances. In day to day management of short-lived illness such as nonspecific gastroenteritis the assessment will be simple and the details of Figure 5.1 may be condensed.

Before starting therapy the patient's weight, height, temperature and blood pressure must be measured and recorded. From these values the maintenance requirements may be calculated. If fever, diarrhoea, polyuria or fistula drainage continues then allowance must be made for modified maintenance therapy. Twice daily clinical examinations and weighing must be done and accurate fluid balance charts kept and reviewed.

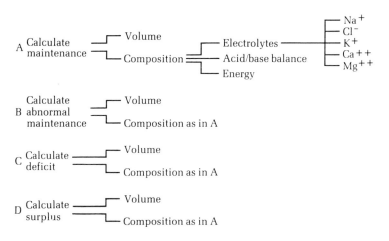

Figure 5.1 Scheme for managing water and electrolyte disorders. The requirements per unit time = A + B + C – D (applies to each constituent of volume and composition).

Maintenance requirements were discussed in Chapter 4; this chapter presents the calculations for deficit and surplus.

Calculation of deficit

Volume — dehydration

Pure water loss is uncommon; the term dehydration customarily means loss of water and sodium. The reduction of fluid volume is distributed throughout the ECF and ICF to a degree proportional to the respective sizes of the ECF and ICF.

Three types of dehydration are recognized in paediatrics: isotonic, hypertonic and hypotonic. In isotonic dehydration water and sodium are lost in equivalent amounts, hypertonic dehydration results from a greater loss of water than sodium, and hypotonic dehydration occurs when sodium loss exceeds fluid loss.

Isotonic dehydration

This may be caused by excessive loss of water and sodium, or inadequate intake — see Table 5.1.

Table 5.1   Causes of isotonic dehydration

Excess output	Deficient intake
Gastrointestinal	Coma
vomiting	Fluid restriction
diarrhoea	
fistulae	
suction	
Insensible loss	
sweat	
Kidney	
solute dependent — diabetes mellitus	
obligatory — diabetes insipidus	
renal tubular disorders	

Effects — clinical: Three stages of dehydration are used, based on loss of weight and are shown in Table 5.2. They are losses of 5%, 10% and 10–15% which correspond to water losses of 50 ml/kg, 100

Table 5.2 Signs of water depletion

% BW lost	Signs
5	Dry mucus membranes; reduced skin turgor; sunken eyeballs; absence of tears and spittle
10	Ill child; low urine output; thirst; poor skin circulation
10-15	Shock; thready, rapid pulse; low blood pressure; anuria; depression of consciousness; hyperventilation

ml/kg and 100–150 ml/kg body weight respectively (in fact as the body water is 65% of body weight these losses are strictly 7.5%, 15% and 15–22.5% of body water). Dehydration greater than 15% is rarely compatible with life.

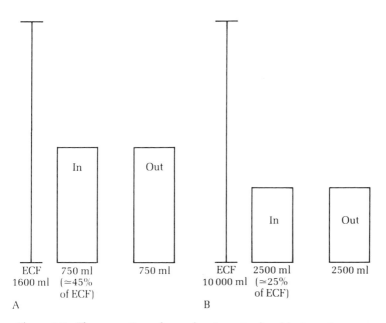

Figure 5.2 The respective volume of water gained and lost per day compared with the ECF volume (not to scale). A. For an infant weighing 5 kg. B. For a teenager weighing 50 kg.

Effects — physiological: Figure 5.2 illustrates the reason why infants are particularly vulnerable to dehydration; the normal daily intake and output of fluid is nearly 50% of the ECF volume in a 5 kg infant, whereas in a 50 kg adolescent they represent about 25% of the ECF volume. Loss of 250 ml fluid is 10% dehydration in a 2.5 kg baby. If oral or intravenous compensation for isotonic loss does not occur certain internal compensations are made. In the kidney the urine volume is reduced due to a reduction in glomerular filtration, the secretion of aldosterone and antidiuretic hormone (ADH), and by volume receptor stimulation. The urine concentration is also increased to levels over 1000 mmol/kg. If dehydration is severe and prolonged the renal circulation may become compromised and acute renal failure supervene. The other compensation is an inter-compartmental shift of water from the ICF to ECF, resulting in contraction of both these compartments until the osmolalities of ECF and ICF are similar.

Laboratory tests are of limited value; the haematocrit may rise but sodium, chloride, potassium and urea levels are unaltered. If there is circulatory impairment in severe dehydration uraemia, hyperkalaemia and metabolic acidosis develop. The urine will be scanty, concentrated to more than $2 \times$ plasma osmolality, but will contain little sodium if aldosterone secretion is normal. If acute tubular necrosis occurs the urine sodium will rise to > 20 mmol/l and the urine urea and osmolality will fall.

Treatment: The fluid deficit should be estimated and should be replaced along with maintenance and abnormal maintenance requirements. Losses should not just be replaced with water as there

Table 5.3 Composition of some oral fluids used in rehydration

	Darrow's solution (50% strength with 2.5% dextrose)	Hartmann's solution (50% strength)
Na	60	65
K	18	2.5
Cl	52	55
Bicarbonate	25 (lactate)	15 (lactate)
Glucose	25 g (136 mmol/l)	—

is invariably some electrolyte loss also. It is customary in the UK to use a small number of replacement fluids to encourage familiarity of use.

Oral rehydration: Dioralyte powder (see Table 4.3) dissolved in tap water (1 sachet to 200 ml water) has taken some of the uncertainty and risk from the traditional prescription of 'sugar and salt' water. Other oral fluids used are 50% strength Hartmann's solution, 50% strength Darrow's/2.5% dextrose (Table 5.3) or, for very short periods, 0.18% saline/4.3% dextrose (see Table 4.4). Standard oral rehydration salts (ORS) contain sodium, potassium citrate (more stable than bicarbonate) and glucose and are widely used in tropical climates. The most widely used salts contain 90 mmol Na/litre and can be used in more temperate climates.

For maintenance a solution containing 30–60 mmol Na/litre should be substituted, or the patient given ORS:water in 2:1 ratio. The amount given is 50 ml/kg (in 5% dehydration) using the initial body weight and accepting that this will be an under correction. This should be replaced over the first 12 hours in addition to maintenance requirements and abnormal maintenance requirements, for example from continuing loss in diarrhoea. Allow 10 ml/kg/24 hours for stool loss when watery diarrhoea continues, and as electrolyte loss also occurs this volume should be replaced with 0.18% saline/4.3% dextrose.

Intravenous rehydration: If oral fluids are not retained or there is severe dehydration then intravenous fluid must be given. With circulatory collapse plasma or physiological saline should be given as a resuscitation fluid in a volume of 10–20 ml/kg in 30 minutes. When large volume deficits are being replaced the body weight and fluid output must be watched closely in case renal insufficiency causes fluid retention and jeopardizes the circulation. Progress must be reviewed no longer than six-hourly.

Hypertonic dehydration

This occurs most commonly when there is greater loss of (hypotonic) water than sodium. The cause is usually diarrhoea occurring in a baby previously given excessively concentrated feeds. Rarely, it results from the inadvertent (or deliberate) administration of excessive salt in home-made glucose saline solutions, diabetes insipidus, hyperosmolar diabetic coma or inadequate water intake in a comatose patient.

Effects — clinical: There is usually a short prodrome of diarrhoea or respiratory symptoms following which the baby becomes lethargic but irritable when roused. The skin consistency is firm and doughy rather than the loose appearance and feel in isotonic dehydration. If fluid loss continues then circulatory collapse occurs abruptly, often without the progression through the physical signs of dehydration. Neurological symptoms are prominent, sometimes mimicking meningitis, and convulsions may complicate hypertonic dehydration before or during treatment. In babies dying during treatment of the condition there is often cerebral oedema with or without haemorrhage or subdural effusions. Hypertonic dehydration was a common cause of death or disability in survivors in the UK until infant feeding practices changed in the mid 1970s. Table 5.4 compares the physical signs in various forms of dehydration.

Table 5.4 Physical signs in dehydration

	Hypotonic or isotonic	Hypertonic
Skin turgor	Lost	Normal until late stage
Skin consistency	Soft	Hard and doughy
Fontanelle	Depressed	Normal or raised
Eyeball tension	Lost	Normal
Peripheral circulation	Poor	Preserved until late stage
Blood pressure	Low	Normal until late stage
Neurological	Not pronounced until late stage	Prominent in early stage

Effects — physiological: Excess loss of water over sodium through the passage of frequent hypotonic stools or in severe respiratory illness, leads to a distortion of the sodium/water relationship. Continued feeding with hypertonic solutions interferes with compensatory renal conservation of water as the solute in the feeds will require water for excretion. These patients usually have a fever leading to further fluid loss from lungs and skin. The effect of this greater loss of water than solute is to make the plasma more concentrated, that is hypertonic or hypernatraemic. When the plasma sodium rises above 150 mmol/l neurological complications become more likely. Since fluid moves more rapidly than solute between body compartments, water will be attracted from the ICF to the ECF in an attempt to dilute the hypertonic ECF and intracellular dehydration will occur — particularly damaging to the cells of the CNS.

Other laboratory findings in hypertonic dehydration are raised plasma potassium (reflecting prerenal failure from hypovolaemia) and glucose, a low pH, and bicarbonate from metabolic acidosis, again probably because of poor renal function. The plasma calcium is often low and this may contribute to the convulsive complications of hypertonic dehydration.

Treatment: The aim is the restoration of ECF and ICF water and osmolality. It is quite clear that if this is done too speedily and with hypotonic fluids severe and often permanent neurological complications will occur. There are several possible mechanisms; hypotonic fluid may quickly pass into dehydrated brain cells causing them to rapidly expand. The cells have a means of compensating for hypernatraemia by generating idiogenic osmoles from peptide breakdown. These seem to make the neural cells particularly vulnerable to rapid influx of water causing cerebral oedema. The intracranial dehydration causes brain shrinkage and rupture of blood vessels. The principle to follow is that, providing the circulatory blood volume and, therefore, renal function can be maintained, then endogenous homeostatic mechanisms will deal with the gross osmolar imbalance.

Several regimes have been suggested; an example is shown in

Table 5.5 Treatment of hypertonic dehydration in a child less than one year old

---

1 If circulatory failure presents administer 20 ml/kg plasma intravenously

2 With intact circulation give 0.18% saline in 4.3% dextrose 100 ml/kg admission weight/24 hours; if infant will tolerate oral fluids give oral electrolyte solution and reduce intravenous infusion volume accordingly

3 Potassium chloride 20 mmol/l should be added to infusion fluid once a satisfactory urine flow is achieved (e.g. 0.5 ml/kg/hour)

4 If circulatory failure and hypotension persist and there is a metabolic acidosis consider half correction with sodium bicarbonate

5 Calcium gluconate infusion (10 ml 10% solution) may be required for symptomatic hypocalcaemia

---

Table 5.5. It will be seen that replacement of deficit is ignored in this regime and a modest maintenance volume supplied. If uncontrollable losses continue then the infusion rate may need to be increased. If the patient has a satisfactory circulation, is not vomiting and will take oral fluids then this route is satisfactory. Various authors have used prophylactic anticonvulsant (phenobarbitone) therapy or dexamethasone administration to reduce cerebral oedema.

Hypotonic dehydration

Here there is either a greater loss of sodium than water or a replacement of isotonic loss with insufficient sodium. The plasma sodium concentration falls; below 130 mmol/l a state of hyponatraemia exists.

Effects — clinical: When there is accompanying water loss there is quick progression to hypotensive dehydration with its characteristic physical signs. As the plasma sodium falls neurological symptoms such as confusion, anxiety, convulsions and depressed level of consciousness occur. Tendon reflexes may be reduced.

Effects — physiological: With the decline in plasma sodium, the plasma osmolality falls also. The ICF is then at a greater osmolality than the ECF, and fluid shifts into the cells causing a reduction in circulating blood volume and hypotension. In the absence of dehydration, fluid will not be readily excreted and the waterlogged patient may develop an encephalopathy.

Treatment: If the patient is shocked then intravenous physiological saline (0.9%) or plasma should be given; a central venous pressure line will help in management. When the circulation is restored and urine is flowing 0.45% saline and dextrose are given to replenish the sodium deficit, and then 0.18% saline and 4.3% dextrose as maintenance. Potassium supplements will often be required when a urine flow is established.

Hypertonic saline: If there is profound hyponatraemia with neurological symptoms then 3% sodium chloride may be given to correct deficiencies according to the formula: $(130 - \text{plasma Na}^+)$ $0.3 \times \text{kg body weight} = \text{mmol Na}^+$ required (note that 1 ml 3% NaCl = 0.5 mmol Na$^+$).

This correction should be made over 4–6 hours. Hypertonic saline should only be used if there are symptoms: it carries the hazard of sodium overload and circulatory compromise. Asymptomatic hyponatraemia is usually treated by fluid restriction, allowing 50% to 75% daily maintenance requirements.

Composition

Sodium (Table 5.6)

The diagnosis and management of one of the commonest causes of sodium deficit has been covered in the section on dehydration. Hyponatraemia may cause profound neurological disturbance; it may be accompanied by a decreased ECF volume due to loss from the gut, kidney skin, or exudative loss, and will need replacement with physiological saline. Hyponatraemia with normal ECF volume is usually caused by water retention secondary to excessive ADH, glucocorticoid or thyroxine deficiency, or diuretic therapy. Treatment is by water restriction. Hyponatraemia with EDF expansion occurs in liver, cardiac or renal failure; careful use of loop diuretics is indicated.

Table 5.6   Clinical causes of hyponatraemia

---

1 Sodium deficit:
inadequate maintenance supply
sodium loss from the gastrointestinal tract (aspiration, fistula)
excessive uncompensated loss from the kidney:
  recovery from acute tubular necrosis
  adrenogenital syndrome (salt-retaining hormone deficit)
  CNS disease

2 Water excess (dilution):
excessive maintenance volume
water retention in:
  renal disease
  excess antidiuretic hormone

3 Artefactual in the presence of hyperlipidaemia, e.g. diabetes mellitus, nephrotic syndrome (Figure 1.3)

Potassium

With an intracellular ion, potassium balance is difficult to assess by clinical or routine laboratory methods. Plasma potassium levels are a poor indication of ICF and therefore of total body potassium states. For practical management the changes in ECF potassium — the plasma potassium — need to be considered. A low serum potassium means depletion of total body potassium. In conditions such as renal failure the plasma potassium may be high with a reduced ICF potassium. Hypokalaemia usually results from uncompensated gastrointestinal or renal loss of potassium (Table 5.7).

Table 5.7 Causes of hypokalaemia

---

1 Gastrointestinal:
vomiting, diarrhoea, fistulae — all contain *c.* 10 mmol K^+/l
2 Renal:
metabolic alkalosis, aldosteronism, diuretic therapy, renal tubular disorders (Fanconi syndrome, Bartter's syndrome)
3 Metabolic:
diabetes mellitus (see Chapter 7)

Effects — clinical: There is usually a history of a condition such as profound diarrhoea or diuretic therapy causing potassium loss. Muscle weakness, diminished tendon reflexes and abdominal distension with few bowel sounds all suggest hypokalaemia. Chronic hypokalaemia affects renal concentrating ability causing polyuria, which may allow further deterioration in renal function in the patient with chronic renal insufficiency. Hypokalaemia causes the electrocardiographic anomalies seen in Table 2.3; cardiac arrhythmias may also occur.

Effects — physiological: Intracellular K^+ deficiency affects cell function particularly in muscle and the brain, causing muscle weakness and alterations of mental state.

Treatment: Potassium should be replaced by mouth either as fruit juice or potassium chloride solutions (which children often find unpalatable). If oral replenishment cannot be done then potassium should be given parenterally — usually intravenously. The potential hazard is elevation of the plasma potassium to toxic levels causing cardiac arrhythmias and arrest. For this reason the potassium concentration of intravenous fluid solutions should only exceed 40 mmol/l in the most exceptional circumstances, and the total daily allowance should be less than 3 mmol/kg. In the severely fluid-depleted child potassium supplements are given once an adequate urine flow is achieved. In practice the contents of an ampoule containing 20 mmol of KCL is added to a litre infusion bag *and well shaken*, and the infusion rate is based on the degree of fluid volume required — so long as renal function is normal and there are no major continuing losses of potassium. If potassium loss continues, for example from a fistula, then much greater amounts of potassium will need to be infused — perhaps up to 10 mmol/kg/24 hours. Serial plasma potassium measurements are required and reliable ECG monitoring is helpful.

Calcium

Conditions affecting bone, kidney, parathyroid or gut functions may cause hypocalcaemia and it often occurs in alkalosis, dehydration, or acute renal failure. In the latter cases the mechanism is obscure, but the control of calcium metabolism in bone is known to be affected by the concentrations of sodium and potassium and abnormal concentrations of these ions may contribute to hypocalcaemia.

Effects — clinical and physiological: Neuromuscular irritability occurs with tetany, muscle twitching and convulsions.

Treatment: Infusion of 10% calcium gluconate 2 ml/kg (0.45 mmol/kg) at not more than 1 ml/minute will relieve acute symptoms. Care must be taken to avoid bradycardia by stopping the injection if the heart rate falls below 80/minute. With prolonged hypocalcaemia infusions may be required with doses up to 1.2 mmol/kg/24 hours. Calcium salts can cause local necrosis if extravasated from the vein, so pump infusions are hazardous. If calcium can be tolerated by mouth, suitable preparations are calcium lactate 300 mg tablets, and in infancy Calcium-Sandoz elixir or calcium glubionate (325 mg calcium (8.1 mmol Ca^{++}) per 15 ml).

Magnesium

Like potassium this is an intracellular ion and plasma levels do not acurately reflect the total body magnesium level. However, unless renal failure is present, depletion of magnesium stores causes a low plasma magnesium level.

Hypomagnasaemia is found in a number of gastrointestinal, renal and metabolic conditions (hyperaldosteronism and parathyroid disorders). The level may fall acutely in dehydration but rarely enough to cause clinical problems. The level should be determined if calcium-resistant tetany or seizures occur. Treatment is magnesium sulphate 0.1 ml/kg of 25% solution intramuscularly 6-hourly or up to 10 ml/kg of a 1% solution by slow intravenous infusion.

Chloride

For clinical purposes chloride may be viewed as a close partner of sodium and that disorders such as hyponatraemic dehydration will cause hypochloraemia. This is also seen in pyloric stenosis where deficiency of chloride in glomerular filtrate impedes sodium reabsorption in the proximal tubule; Na^+ is therefore exchanged for K^+ and H^+ in the distal tubule, giving an acid urine and perpetuating the alkalotic state. Treatment of hypochloraemia is by giving chloride salts of sodium and, to a lesser extent, potassium in treatment of the cation deficiency. Sometimes the chloride level remains low with neurological weakness despite administration of generous amounts of isotonic saline. Ammonium chloride salt is used, but only when plasma volume is restored.

Hydrogen ion — alkalosis

The complex controls of acid/base balance have been dealt with in Chapter 3. A deficit in hydrogen ion may be caused by metabolic or respiratory disorders, or a combination of both.

Metabolic alkalosis: This arises from loss of H^+, most commonly from the stomach in pyloric stenosis; otherwise it is a consequence of diuretic therapy or some rare metabolic conditions such as aldosteronism. The main effect is tetany caused by the change of calcium from ionized to the bound form. There is a rise in the plasma bicarbonate level. Treatment is rarely required; if symptoms such as respiratory depression occur then ammonium chloride can be given.

Respiratory alkalosis: This does not need specific therapy as it usually arises from hyperventilation, and the primary cause of this should be treated. Respiratory alkalosis is sometimes deliberately induced, for instance in the management of cerebral oedema.

Energy

In short illnesses energy deficit is not a pressing clinical concern. If protracted deficiency occurs then convalescence will be delayed. In these circumstances nutrition should be given by tube feeding or parenterally; the topic is discussed further in Chapter 11.

Calculation of surplus

Volume — water

Overhydration occurs when the amount of fluid taken in is consistently greater than the amount lost in urine, sweat, faeces and from the lungs.

Effects — clinical and physiological

There is usually dependant oedema — particularly if there is isotonic overhydration with salt and water. In severe cases the plasma volume will expand and cause hypertension and heart failure.

Treatment

This is a condition which must be avoided by careful attention to fluid balance charts and body weight. Particular care must be taken where fluids are given in the face of dehydration and poor urine flow. If the kidneys are functioning normally then fluid intake should be cut back to allow excretion of excess fluid. If there is raised blood pressure or signs of myocardial dysfunction then, frusemide 1 mg/kg should be given. When there is renal insufficiency, fluid overload is an indication for dialysis.

Syndrome of inappropriate antidiuretic hormone secretion (SIADH) (see Chapter 10)

This is the name given to the condition commonly seen in cerebral and other disorders, where oliguria occurs despite normal renal function and adequate fluid status. Water is retained and dilutional hyponatraemia occurs.

Composition

Sodium and chloride

Although there may appear to be an excess of sodium and chloride in hypernatraemic dehydration this is really due to water deficit. True sodium and chloride excess results from poisoning — either by inadvertently mistaking salt for sugar, or by administration of salt solutions as an emetic in accidental poisoning. Cases of malicious poisoning have been recorded.

The treatment is similar to that for hypertonic dehydration — cautious administration of maintenance fluid. Diuretic therapy (frusemide, bumetanide) has been used, and the severely intoxicated and symptomatic child might best be managed by peritoneal dialysis. In certain metabolic disorders, such as renal tubular acidosis, there is a fall in bicarbonate with a compensatory rise in chloride. Again, the treatment is of the primary condition.

Potassium

Hyperkalaemia occurs if there is poor excretion, as in renal failure or acidosis, or if there is excessive tissue breakdown, such as seen in therapy of malignant disease. Unfortunately some cases of potassium intoxication are caused by the prescription of excessive amounts in therapy.

Effects — clinical and physiological: Very high ($\geqslant$ 8 mmol/l) levels of potassium compromise muscle function; skeletal muscle weakness and cardiac arrhythmias or arrest occurs. Table 2.3 shows the electrocardiograph changes in hyperkalaemia.

Treatment: There are four complementary methods of treating this medical emergency:

1 Expand the ECF to dilute the plasma potassium: use intravenous physiological saline 10 ml/kg or sodium bicarbonate 1 mmol/kg.

2 Antagonizing effects of K^+ on muscle membrane: use calcium gluconate 10% solution 0.5 ml/kg by slow intravenous injection.

3 Increase the cellular uptake of K^+: use intravenous glucose 0.5 g/kg. Non-diabetics metabolize this within an hour. Insulin is not really necessary but 0.1 unit of soluble insulin/kg body weight is sometimes given intravenously with the glucose.

4 Remove K^+ from the body:

(a) by oral or rectal resins such as calcium resonium 1 g/kg/24 hours;

(b) by diuretics such as frusemide 1 mg/kg, or more;

(c) by dialysis.

Calcium

Hypercalcaemia is not a recognized complication of fluid balance disorders. However it may itself cause derangement of the body fluids. It is caused by vitamin D intoxication, hyperparathyroidism and malignancy.

Effects — clinical and physiological: Microscopic calcium deposition in the kidney interferes with renal concentrating ability. If this is longstanding then the changes will be permanent. Polyuria occurs, and if this is not compensated by an adequate fluid intake dehydration will occur. Other effects of hypercalcaemia are depression of tendon reflexes and ECG (electrocardiograph) changes — shortening of the Q-T interval and sinus bradycardia.

Treatment (see Chapter 10):

1 Reduce intake of vitamin D and calcium.

2 Restore circulating fluid volume.

3 Promote calcium excretion with diuretics such as frusemide.

4 Phosphates.

5 Prednisolone (not usually effective in hyperparathyroidism).

6 Calcitonin.

Magnesium

This most commonly occurs in renal failure or as a complication of magnesium therapy.

Effects — clinical and physiological: Magnesium is concerned with nervous function. Hypermagnesaemia causes coma, and depressed reflexes and respiration.

Treatment: Treat with intravenous calcium gluconate; in renal failure dialysis will be required.

Hydrogen ion — acidosis

Accumulation of H$^+$ occurs rarely from excess intake, or more commonly from diminished excretion in renal tubular acidosis, or renal failure. Excessive endogenous production will result from states of shock, anoxia, diabetic ketoacidosis and poor tissue perfusion.

Effects — clinical: Hyperventilation occurs as a compensatory measure to lower Pco_2 and limit the fall in pH. The deep, sighing respirations are known as Kussmaul breathing. Vascular resistance and cardiac function fall and there is tissue hypoxia, drowsiness and coma.

Treatment: This must be directed to the primary cause — limiting production of ketoacids in diabetes by giving fluid and insulin, and promoting the excretion of drugs or poisons such as salicylic acid. In chronic conditions, such as primary renal tubular acidosis, alkali is the main treatment. Its use is more controversial in acute metabolic acidosis because of concern about inducing alkalaemia and causing a further fall in intracellular pH. In diabetic ketoacidosis bicarbonate therapy may cause a profound fall in serum potassium and special care must be taken. If bicarbonate is given then the formula for dosage should be that given on p.32. Bicarbonate therapy should be diluted and the correction made every 4–6 hours. It must be emphasized that in most patients with acute metabolic acidosis and who previously had normal kidneys, treatment of the primary cause plus fluid and electrolyte replacement is usually sufficient. There is no merit in very rapid correction — once shock is corrected.

Respiratory acidosis: The primary event is poor respiratory gaseous exchange and CO_2 retention leading to accumulation of H$^+$. There is often a metabolic component since hypoxia and anaerobic metabolism results in the production of lactic acid in the ECF. The treatment is to restore ventilation. Alkali therapy plays no part.

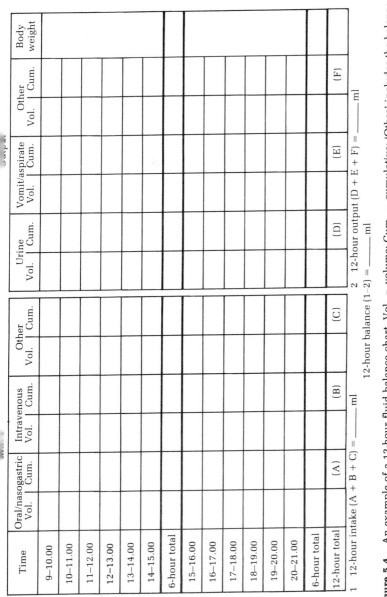

Time	Oral/nasogastric Vol.	Cum.	Intravenous Vol.	Cum.	Other Vol.	Cum.	Urine Vol.	Cum.	Vomit/aspirate Vol.	Cum.	Other Vol.	Cum.	Body weight
9–10.00													
10–11.00													
11–12.00													
12–13.00													
13–14.00													
14–15.00													
6-hour total													
15–16.00													
16–17.00													
17–18.00													
18–19.00													
19–20.00													
20–21.00													
6-hour total													
12-hour total	(A)		(B)		(C)		(D)		(E)		(F)		

1 12-hour intake (A + B + C) = _____ ml

2 12-hour output (D + E + F) = _____ ml

12-hour balance (1–2) = _____ ml

Figure 5.4. An example of a 12-hour fluid balance chart. Vol. = volume; Cum. = cumulative; 'Other' includes the balance of peritoneal dialysis exchanges.

Conclusion

From the foregoing a unified scheme for treating water and electrolyte problems can be constructed and applied to any clinical disorders. The framework is the same whatever condition is being treated, be it burns or gastroenteritis and dehydration. Figure 5.4 shows a 12-hour fluid balance chart that may be used for straightforward problems. In cases such as renal failure 4–6 hourly calculations of electrolyte intake and output may be required. Separate charts for other aspects of fluid balance will be required — such as for peritoneal dialysis. When nutrition is poor for a prolonged period then an accurate intake chart is required for energy, carbohydrate, protein and fat to compare with desirable intakes.

Clinical Aspects

6

Gastroenteritis, Dehydration and Shock

Gastroenteritis and dehydration

The commonest cause of acute fluid and electrolyte derangement throughout the world is infection of the gastrointestinal tract. In countries where infant malnutrition is widespread such infections cause millions of deaths, but the last 50 years have seen an encouraging decline in mortality in the UK.

Causes

The infective agent will depend on the part of the world where the child lives. In the UK in children under two years old *Rotavirus* and specific *Escherichia coli* infections are common, but in some cases no organism can be identified (nonspecific diarrhoea). Over the age of two a bacterial cause is more likely; examples are *Shigella*, *Salmonella* and *Campylobacter* species.

Effects

Vomiting and diarrhoea immediately upset fluid and electrolyte balance because of deficient intake and excessive loss. Energy intake will be reduced and body stores (carbohydrate, fat and protein) will be drawn upon. In a minor 24-hour episode, providing sufficient water is offered, renal compensatory mechanisms will ameliorate losses and the short period of poor nutrition will be inconsequential. If the losses are greater, or continue for longer, the extracellular volume (ECV) will contract despite some repletion from the ICF; plasma volume and glomerular filtration will decline, and hydrogen ion produced from catabolism will not be excreted and metabolic acidosis will ensue. The compensatory hyperventilation (Kussmaul respiration) will increase insensible fluid loss.

In most cases of gastroenteritis sodium and water are lost in equivalent amounts resulting in isotonic dehydration. If attempts at

67

rehydration result in an intake of water greater than sodium for more than 24 hours then the serum sodium will fall and hypotonic dehydration will result. In infants who have customarily been given milk formula feeds containing excessive sodium and whose hypertonic feeds are continued in the face of excess loss and inadequate replenishment, hypertonic (hypernatraemic) dehydration follows. Clinical descriptions are given in Chapter 4.

Treatment

Short-lived mild symptoms

Most healthy and well nourished infants and children will come to no harm providing feeds are withdrawn. Time-honoured remedies such as adding pinches of salt to water should be avoided. Plain tap water will suffice for rehydration lasting a few hours. When electrolytes are required an oral glucose-electrolyte mixture (or Oral Rehydration Salts — citrate, WHO) such as Dioralyte should be prescribed. Errors in reconstitution may occur so it is wise to have it prepared in a pharmacy. In infants less than one year old, volumes of 150 ml/kg/24 hours are ideal, but it is wise to start with frequent small volumes (e.g 1.5 ml/kg/hour, each hour) and gradually increase according to the child's tolerance. When symptoms have stopped and clear fluids absorbed then it is traditional to regrade feed intake using 25%, 50% and 75% strength milk over 48–72 hours. In most cases this can be done more quickly — indeed some paediatricians question whether any regrading is necessary and that it merely prolongs malnutrition. Toddlers who are weaned can progress from milk to solids — usually according to preference rather than suitability.

Major dehydration

Children who are 5% dehydrated or more require hospital admission.
Observations should include:
1 Weight and blood pressure on admission and daily thereafter until symptoms abate.
2 Intake and output chart.
3 Plasma urea and electrolyte measurements.

Fluids and electrolytes: If the circulation is stable one or two attempts at frequent, small volume, clear fluid replacement may be made and if this is not vomited management proceeds as in the mild case. Where vomiting continues or the stool volume outstrips the replacement volume, dehydration will progress and intravenous therapy is needed. Patients who are 10% dehydrated require immediate intravenous therapy for restoring blood volume and flow deficit.

The fluid composition for the treatment of isotonic dehydration is shown in Table 6.1. Notice that it conforms to the blueprint of treatment shown in Chapter 5. In cases of severe dehydration a raised blood urea is often seen. This is usually caused by hypovolaemic pre-renal failure, and fluid replacement re-establishes urine formation and a fall in blood urea. If this does not happen then either fluid replacement has not been sufficient or acute intrinsic renal failure may have supervened and fluid restriction may be necessary (see Chapter 8). Intravenous fluid therapy is continued until vomiting ceases and oral glucose-electrolyte or water can be recommended; when these are tolerated milk may be given.

Specific therapy: Anti-emetic and antidiarrhoeal drugs are still prescribed for acute intestinal upsets in children but there is no evidence that they influence the severity or duration of the disorder.

Since the majority of childhood gastroenteritis is caused by viruses, antibiotics have no place in management. The current indications for antibiotic use are:

1 Septicaemia with bacterial gastroenteritis, such as *Salmonella typh* infection.
2 *Campylobacter* infection. This often has a very acute onset with severe abdominal pain and bloody diarrhoea. If these organisms are isolated and symptoms continue then a course of oral erythromycin should be given (though erythromycin sometimes causes abdominal pain and nausea).
3 Colonization with *Giardia lamblia* — especially in the immuno-deficient child — warrants treatment with metronidazole.

Prevention

Infective gastroenteritis is transmitted from person to person by the faecal–oral route. Scrupulous handwashing and wearing of gowns are used to prevent spread in institutions: if a hospital ward or

Table 6.1 Fluid and electrolyte replacement in gastroenteritis, using as an example a 10 kg child with 10% dehydration after 48 hours diarrhoea

	Volume	Composition
Deficit	10% of 10 kg (1000ml)	Na (25 mmol/l) 25 mmol K (20 mmol/l) 20 mmol Cl (25 mmol/l) 25 mmol
Surplus	none	none
Maintenance	100 × 10 (1000 ml)	Na (2.5 × 10) 25 mmol K (2.5 × 10) 25 mmol Cl (2.5 × 20) 25 mmol
Abnormal maintenance*	100 ml	Na 2.5 mmol K 2.0 mmol Cl 2.5 mmol
Total required in first 24 hours	Water 2100 ml	Na 52.5 mmol K 47 mmol Cl 52.5 mmol
Management Initial therapy (first hour): 0.9% NaCl 10 mg/kg	100 ml	Na 15 mmol K 0 mmol Cl 15 mmol
24 hours i.v. fluid: 0.18% NaCl/4.3% dextrose + 20 mmol/l KCL†	2000	Na 62 mmol K 40 mmol Cl 102 mmol
Total	2100	Na 77 mmol K 40 mmol Cl 117 mmol

Comments:
1 KCl is not added to the infusion until urine is passed.
2 Na^+ and K^+ requirements are approximately met: under- or over-provision will be regulated by renal conservation or excretion.
3 Excessive chloride is given, and is excreted via the kidneys.
4 Energy is ignored. Probably 2520 J/24 hours (600 cal/24 hours) are required but body stores will suffice in the short term. Note that the 0.18% NaCl/4.3% dextrose supplies 1155 J (275 cal) in 24 hours. This will prevent hypoglycaemia but must not be regarded as an adequate single energy source for more than a few days.
5 Calcium, magnesium and phosphate are ignored; body stores will suffice for a short illness.

*Assuming 24 hours continuing diarrhoea of similar composition.
†1000 in next 7 hours, and remaining 1000 ml over the following 16 hours.

nursery has an outbreak of infective gastroenteritis no new admissions are allowed until all infective cases are removed. Most hospitals in the UK have a named member of staff to advise on control of infection.

Prognosis

Most attacks of gastroenteritis are short lived and the child is back to normal within a week. If symptoms recur on reintroduction of milk and solids then temporary lactase deficiency should be suspected; it may be rapidly confirmed by the discovery of reducing substances in the stools. Toddler diarrhoea or the 'currants and peas' syndrome sometimes follows an acute episode of gastroenteritis; children with this condition always thrive despite frequent loose stools containing undigested food. If the child does not thrive then the other conditions shown in Table 6.2 should be considered.

Rarely, acute gastroenteritis is followed by a prolonged period of food intolerance with recurring episodes of diarrhoea. In these circumstances malnutrition may occur so that supplemental nutrition should be considered early, whilst the best absorbed diet can be identified and established.

Shock

Causes

This describes the clinical state of a patient in whom there is either profound reduction of the circulating blood volume (haemorrhage or dehydration), failure of the cardiac pump (cardiogenic shock) or exceptional dilation of the peripheral circulation (septic shock). All three may coexist.

Effects

The symptoms are of syncope, shivering and sweating; the signs are low blood pressure, fast pulse rate, cold extremities with slow refill of capillaries, oliguria and a core–peripheral temperature gap of $>1°C$. Investigations include the measurement of plasma creatinine and electrolytes, determination of acid/base status and blood and other cultures.

Table 6.2 Some causes of recurrent diarrhoea in childhood

Cause	Diagnosis	Management
Lactose intolerance	> 0.5% reducing substance in stool fluid	Temporary withdrawal of lactose from diet
Cow's milk protein (CMP) intolerance	Clinical, using milk challenges	Withdraw CMP
Toddler diarrhoea	By exclusion in a thriving child	None required
Antibiotic diarrhoea	History of repeated courses of antibiotics	Withdraw antibiotics
Giardiasis	Identification of *Giardia lamblia* in stool or jejunal fluid	Metronidazole
Other chronic infective diarrhoea, e.g. amoebiasis	Identity organism	Appropriate chemotherapy
Inflammatory bowel disease	X-rays and biopsy	Anti-inflammatory drugs

Treatment

Management depends on the cause. Pure haemorrhagic shock should be treated by administering oxygen and by blood replacement with 10 ml/kg whole blood over 15–30 minutes. This should be repeated until the blood pressure rises, the peripheral circulation improves, the temperature gap closes, and urine is passed. A central venous pressure (CVP) line helps in management, and transfusion should continue until the CVP is >1330 Pa (10 mmHg).

Dehydration should be managed similarly, but plasma or dextrose are substituted for blood unless the haematocrit is lower than 30%. If the signs of shock have not improved then a cardiogenic element must be suspected. In cardiogenic shock potent cardiac stimulants will be needed; examples are isoprenaline (100 ng/kg/min to a maximum of 1.5 μg/kg/min) and dopamine (2 μg/kg/min increased by 2 μg/kg/min increments to 20 μg/kg/min).

Where it is suspected that peripheral vascular resistance is maintaining shock then peripheral vasodilator therapy should be used. Nitroprusside (1 μg/kg/min increased by 1 μg/kg/min to a maximum of 10 μg/kg/min) is used but only after volume expansion has been effected. Some use high-dose steroids (methylpresnisolone 30 mg/kg/6 hours) in septic shock.

Once the shock is overcome an estimate should be made of water and electrolyte deficit and continuing loss, and this corrected with maintenance therapy which is given at the same time.

7

Diabetes Mellitus

The diabetic child is vulnerable to several emergencies which involve fluid balance: ketoacidosis, hyperosmolar coma and hypoglycaemia. Temporary loss of diabetic control may also occur around the time of operative surgery.

Ketoacidosis

This is a true medical emergency which requires meticulous treatment. Successful management is built on an understanding of the metabolic derangements which follow insulin deficiency. Insulin conserves glucose by storing it as glycogen in liver and muscle. Without insulin glycogen is broken down to provide energy, and when this reserve is exhausted fat and protein are catabolized to free fatty acids and amino acids. Both of these are metabolized to glucose in the liver with the production of the ketone bodies acetone, acetoacetic acid and hydroxybutyrate.

The metabolic consequences of insulin deficiency are therefore:
1 Hyperglycaemia.
2 Dehydration and electrolyte inbalance.
3 Ketoacidosis.
4 Hyperosmolality.

Dehydration results from the osmotic diuresis produced by hyperglycaemia, from vomiting and from increased insensible loss caused by hyperventilation. Sodium and potassium ions are lost in the urine and gastrointestinal tract, and the fluid loss depletes the circulating blood volume causing prerenal insufficiency. A metabolic acidosis results from the accummulation of ketoacids and the fall in H^+ excretion because of poor renal perfusion and function.

Effects

The patient will have a history of polyuria and thirst and will appear dehydrated, confused or comatose, and may have acidotic

Kussmaul respiration. The combination of hyperosmolality, acidosis and shock contribute to coma; rare associated conditions such as meningitis or drug ingestion must not be overlooked. The chief diagnostic traps are confusing diabetic ketoacidosis with pneumonia (particularly in infancy), salicylate poisoning, or renal failure because of the sighing respiratory pattern. Diabetes may mimic an acute abdominal condition as severe abdominal pain is a common early symptom of diabetic ketoacidosis in childhood.

Treatment

In the new patient with glycosuria the diagnosis is rapidly confirmed by a dextrostix or BM-test-glycemie 20-800. A glucose level greater than 10 mmol/l is diagnostic. (The only other common conditions that might mimic diabetic ketoacidosis are a subarachnoid haemorrhage with glycosuria and chronic renal failure with a renal tubular leak of glucose. The history of the former and a normal blood glucose in the latter should settle the point.) The standard form of management of fluid and electrolyte balance should be followed:

1 Weighing.
2 Assessment of the state of hydration.
3 Blood pressure recording.
4 Blood taken for urea, electrolytes and glucose estimations and acid/base studies.

The serum may be lipaemic and the plasma Na^+ concentration may be falsely low (pseudohyponatraemia; see Chapter 1). An intravenous infusion should be started and a nasogastric tube passed.

The principles of management are similar to any other fluid/electrolyte disorder, namely calculation of deficit, maintenance and abnormal maintenance. This takes precedence over any other measure — including insulin — as it is the loss of sodium and water which contribute most to the clinical features of diabetic ketoacidosis. A plan of fluid and electrolyte management is shown in Table 7.1. Four further factors need discussion: insulin therapy, alkali therapy, potassium and phosphate.

Insulin therapy

Insulin therapy in ketoacidosis is given either by continuous infusion or by hourly intramuscular injections of a soluble insulin

Table 7.1 Fluid and electrolyte replacement in diabetic ketoacidosis, using as an example a semicomatose child of 20 kg with Kussmaul breathing (i.e. *c.* 10% dehydrated)

	Volume	Composition
Deficit	10% of 20 kg (2000 ml)	Na 200 mmol K 100 mmol Cl 150 mmol
Surplus	None	None
Maintenance	90* × 20 (1800 mmol)	Na^+ (2 × 20) 40 mmol K^+ (2 × 20) 40 mmol Cl^- (2 × 20) 40 mmol
Abnormal maintenance	Gastric aspirate 200 ml	Na 10 mmol K 3 mmol Cl 25 mmol
Total required in first 24 hours	Water 3800 ml	Na^+ 250 mmol K^+ 143 mmol Cl^- 215 mmol
Management Initial therapy (first hour): 0.9% saline 20 ml/kg + 20 mmol KCl/l	400 ml	Na^+ 60 mmol K^+ 8 mmol Cl^- 68 mmol
In next 7 hours: 0.45% saline/2.5% dextrose + 30 mmol KCl/l	1600 ml	Na^+ 120 mmol K^+ 48 mmol Cl^- 168 mmol
In next 16 hours: (a) 0.18% saline/4.3% dextrose + 30 mmol KCl/l	1800 ml	Na^+ 56 mmol K^+ 54 mmol Cl^- 100 mmol
(b) 0.9% saline + 10 mmol KCl/l gastric aspirate replacement	200 ml	Na^+ 30 mmol K^+ 2 mmol Cl^- 32 mmol
Total	4000 ml	Na^+ 266 mmol K^+ 112 mmol Cl^- 378 mmol

Comments:
1 KCl added to infusion at start because insulin is also given but KCl should be delayed if plasma potassium is high
2 Note that 10% of the replacement and maintenance combined is given in the first hour; and that 5% of the replacement and maintenance combined is given in 8 hours
3 Gastric aspirate cannot be calculated at the outset; the tube is aspirated hourly and replaced volume for volume with intravenous fluid
4 Na^+ and Cl^- are replaced adequately
5 K^+ undercorrected: sufficient to probably maintain plasma K^+ but supplements will need to be continued to replenish body stores

* See Table 4.1.

preparation. There is no place for subcutaneous insulin or longer-acting insulin as absorption will be erratic and the hypoglycaemic actions unpredictable.

Intravenous infusion: First a bolus of soluble insulin 0.2 unit/kg is given, then a syringe is filled with 0.9% saline plus soluble insulin 1 ml to 1 unit and a dose of 0.1 unit/kg/hour infused. This infusion can be into a separate vein from the rehydrating fluids or can be attached to the main infusion line via a three-way tap. It should not be added to the fluid bag of the main infusion. Some authorities recommend that intravenous infusion of insulin should be prepared in albumin rather than saline as the insulin may be absorbed onto plastic syringes and tubing. Intravenous insulin has a half life of less than 5 minutes, so the infusion should not be stopped without providing insulin by some other route as the blood glucose will rise again. If the blood glucose has not fallen by more than 3 mmol/l in 4 hours then the rate of infusion should be doubled. When the blood glucose drops to 10 mmol/l the infusion can be reduced to 0.02 unit/kg/hour until the child is eating and a sliding scale of insulin administration used.

Intramuscular injections: Providing the circulation is stable then hourly intramuscular injections of 0.1 unit/kg soluble insulin will reduce the blood glucose satisfactorily. The dose will need to be reduced when the blood glucose falls to below 10 mmol/l.

The aim of treatment is a smooth reduction in blood glucose with clearing of ketonuria; fluid therapy alone will cause a fall in blood glucose of about 5 mmol/l. There is no advantage to be gained in very rapid changes and there may be undesirable side effects, such as cerebral oedema. The aim should be to reduce the blood glucose by 2.5 mmol/l/hour. When the child has recovered and is taking food either a 6-hour sliding scale (Table 7.2) can be used for subcutaneous soluble insulin dosage, or an empirical 6-hourly dose of 0.2 unit/kg can be given and adjustments made in the light of capillary blood glucose readings. Later the maintenance dose of insulin can be started according to the physician's preference.

Alkali therapy

Patients in ketoacidosis have a profound metabolic acidosis because of the production of ketoacids and the decreased renal clearance of H^+. At very low levels of pH there is a risk of cardiac arrest from

Table 7.2 Sliding scale for urine glucose

Urine glucose (g/100 ml)	Dose of subcutaneous soluble insulin 6-hourly (unit/kg)
5	0.5
2.5	0.4
1	0.3
0.5	0.2
Trace	0.1

depression of myocardial contractility and the left ventricular systolic pressure. Acidosis also interferes with ventilation and gaseous exchange. The logical treatment is to give sodium bicarbonate but this has been criticized because:

1 Sodium bicarbonate dissociates, namely $NaCHO_3 \rightarrow Na^+ + HCO_3^-$ and $HCO_3^- + H^+ \rightarrow H_2O + CO_2$. The CO_2 produced needs to be removed by adequate respiratory effort which may be lacking in a comatose patient.

2 Sodium bicarbonate solutions are hyperosmolar and will accentuate the hyperosmolar state of hyperglycaemia, ketonaemia and uraemia.

3 Bicarbonate interferes with oxygen release from haemoglobin.

4 Carbon dioxide passes more rapidly into the cerebrospinal fluid (CSF) than does bicarbonate; the CSF pH will fall.

These risks and benefits have to be assessed in each case, but if the pH is less than 7.1 on admission and remains so or falls during early rehydration, or if there is hypotension refractory to volume replacement then bicarbonate can be given according to the formula on p. 32. This should be infused over 1 hour and the pH checked an hour later. By this time endogenous bicarbonate should have been generated from ketone oxidation and the pH should be above 7.15. If the pH is unaltered or falling and there is no clinical improvement then a second dose may be given. Once the acidosis is reversed and fluid and electrolyte balance are being restored body compensatory mechanisms will do the rest.

Potassium

Intracellular potassium levels are depleted — particularly in the newly diagnosed diabetic. However, as was discussed in Chapter 2, the plasma level of potassium is a crude and sometimes misleading index of body potassium values. Diabetic ketoacidosis illustrates this point well: in the dehydrated state with poor renal perfusion and acidosis the plasma potassium will probably be high, despite low intracellular levels, because potassium will have leaked out of the cells. With rehydration and insulin therapy (and, perhaps, bicarbonate) the potassium rapidly moves back into the cell with glucose, causing a profound fall in plasma potassium. If the child has been in circulatory collapse for any length of time then intrinsic renal failure, unresponsive to volume replacement, may occur and cause potassium retention. The more likely danger in most cases is of hypokalaemia.

Therefore, providing that the child has not been hypotensive and insulin therapy has started, potassium may be given in the rehydrating fluid. If in any doubt it should be withheld until urine is voided. Oral potassium supplements may be required for several days after treatment.

Phosphate

The rapid return of glucose and potassium to the cells is accompanied by intracellular migration of phosphate as glycogen is formed. The plasma phosphate will fall: this is of doubtful clinical significance in the short term, but some recommend the administration of part of the potassium as phosphate salt (K_2HPO_4/KH_2PO_4). The plasma calcium may also fall asymptomatically.

Non-ketotic hyperosmolar coma

This is rarer than ketoacidosis in children, and its cause is not known. There is rapidly progressive dehydration with marked hyperglycaemia and hyperosmolality. The complications are neurological, with fits and coma, and vascular with arterial thrombosis. The mortality and morbidity are high. Treatment is similar to that for hypernatraemia with slow rehydration once the circulation is restored, and low-dose infusion of insulin 0.02 unit/kg/hour.

Hypoglycaemia

This usually occurs following unexpected exercise, a delay in feeding, or a mistake in insulin dosage. The treatment is to abort the attack with oral glucose; if this is insufficient and neurological symptoms occur then glucagon 1 mg is given intramuscularly. When the child arrives at hospital glucose 1 g/kg as 25% solution (50% diluted 1:1 with sterile water) is given intravenously, and a 10% dextrose infusion set up if a long-acting insulin has been given in the last 12 hours. If in doubt about the cause of coma in a diabetic child an infusion of glucose should be given.

Surgery and the diabetic child

There should be as much preparation as possible — even for the most minor procedure. The major hazard is of unrecognized hypoglycaemia occurring during anaesthesia with resulting brain injury. Hyperglycaemia is less immediately dangerous but may progress to ketoacidosis with its own complications. Emergency surgery should be delayed if at all feasible until the patient is acceptably rehydrated, the acid/base status adjusted, and the blood glucose less than 10 mmol/l.

Procedure

Pre-operative

1 Some physicians admit the child at least 24 hours before surgery and give soluble insulin on a thrice daily sliding scale regime (Table 7.2). A profile of blood glucose results may be obtained using BM 20-800 sticks.
2 The child should be fasted according to the anaesthetist's policy.
3 Before going to theatre an infusion of 5% dextrose should be started to avoid ketosis.
4 An infusion of insulin (as described in the section on keto-acidosis) should be set up to run at 0.02 unit/kg/hour.

Intra-operative

5 A sampling venous line should be established (away from the glucose and insulin lines) and regular samples tested on BM 20-800 sticks.
6 The insulin infusion rate should be varied to control the blood glucose between 5–10 mmol/l.

Postoperative

7 Intravenous infusions of glucose and insulin (with maintenance requirements of sodium and potassium) should continue until oral feeding is established when the sliding scale using urine or blood glucose may be reintroduced.

8 If there is major surgery and no nutrition for several days, insulin requirements will increase and potassium and phosphate supplements will be needed.

8

Kidney Disease

Acute renal failure

When a previously healthy patient abruptly loses the excretory function of the kidneys the condition is called acute renal failure (ARF). The most common — but not invariable — symptom is a reduced urine output. This is sometimes not recognized until the renal failure has become symptomatic and, therefore, children who have conditions which predispose to ARF should have their fluid balance charts and weights carefully monitored.

Acute renal failure can be conveniently divided into three physiological and anatomical levels. Table 8.1 shows these levels and some aetiological factors: the common end point is a reduction in the volume of plasma filtered at the glomerulus. The history will give the cause of acute renal failure in most cases but sometimes specialized X-rays, ultrasound, and isotope studies are required. A renal biopsy may help in diagnosing the cause of intrinsic renal failure and a urologist may need to perform an endoscopy. Such investigations are usually deferred until the child has had the immediate fluid disorder dealt with.

One important distinction to be made is between advanced prerenal failure in a shocked child and intrinsic renal failure following hypovolaemic ischaemic damage to the kidneys. Microscopic and chemical examination of the urine will help in this and it is justifiable to pass a catheter into the bladder to obtain a specimen. This manoeuvre will also exclude urethral obstruction and acute retention as causes of oliguria. The catheter should then be removed in case it causes infection or urethral damage. Table 8.2 shows the results of the investigations; there is inevitably some overlap and the clinical findings must be taken into account. Interpretation of these results is especially difficult in the newborn, if diuretics have been used, or if there is chronic renal disease.

Table 8.1 Levels, causes and treatment of acute renal failure

Level	Causes	Treatment
Prerenal	Hypovolaemia from dehydration, blood loss, burns, cardiac failure, or diuretic therapy in renal or liver disease	1 Anticipate volume loss 2 Replace fluid volume 3 Frusemide 4 Anticipate progression to intrinsic renal failure — acute tubular necrosis
Renal (intrinsic)	Renal parenchymal disease from acute tubular necrosis, glomerulonephritis, haemolytic-uraemic syndrome, drugs, acute pyelonephritis (especially infants), renal vein thrombosis, renal cortical necrosis, or urate or calcium nephropathy in malignant disease	1 Treat any amenable primary cause 2 Water and electrolyte control 3 Nutrition 4 Dialysis
Postrenal	Outflow obstruction — neoplastic Ureteric obstruction — calculus in single kidney Vesico-ureteric obstruction — postoperatively, uretercoele(s) Urethral obstruction — valves calculus	1 Restore metabolic equilibrium 2 Surgery

Table 8.2 Differentiation of causes of acute renal failure on a random sample of urine

	Prerenal	Renal
Urine sediment	Normal or few casts	Casts, fragmented red cells
Urine/plasma ratio of creatinine or urea	>10	<10
Urine Na$^+$ concentration	<10 mmol/l	>20 mmol/l
Fractional excretion of Na$^+$*	<1%	>1%
Urine/plasma osmolality ratio	>1.3	<1.1

*Fractional excretion of sodium =

$$\frac{(\text{urine Na mmol/l}) / (\text{plasma Na mmol/l})}{(\text{urine creatinine } \mu\text{mol/l}) / (\text{plasma creatinine } \mu\text{mol/l})} \times 100$$

This is a measure of tubular ability to reabsorb Na$^+$. In hypovolaemic states very little Na$^+$ should be excreted if the renin/angiotensin/ aldosterone system and the renal tubules are functioning normally.

Effects

Fluid balance

Most children with ARF are oliguric. One definition of this is a urine output of less than 300 ml/m^{2}24 hours; another is a urine flow of less than 0.5 ml/kg/hour. However it is possible for a child to be passing large volumes of urine and still have urea and potassium retention. Once oliguria is recognized as not being due to fluid depletion then fluid intake from all sources must be restricted and an accurate balance chart kept and the child weighed twice daily.

Plasma electrolytes will be variably affected; the sodium and chloride will often be normal but occasionally reduced when there is lipaemia (see p. 6) or antecedent vomiting replaced by water only. The plasma potassium will rise and, if this cannot be controlled, dialysis will be required to prevent life-threatening cardiac arrhythmias. Hydrogen ion excretion will decline and a metabolic acidosis will result. This may be helpful if the potassium is raised, since the acidosis will increase the proportion of ionized calcium in the plasma and decrease the excitability of the cardiac cell membrane (but care will need to be taken if the acidosis is treated with bicarbonate). Phosphate will also be retained and the serum calcium will fall; these do not have major implications in the short term and are better left uncorrected. The excretion of urea and creatinine is inadequate; however uraemia is rarely life threatening, but when severe it causes neurological depression and vomiting which will interfere with nutritional intake.

Clinical

In prerenal failure the previously described signs of dehydration will be present with loss of skin turgor, hypotension and tachycardia. With intrinsic renal failure the patient or parents will notice a falling urinary output and, if intake is maintained, oedema will form in the face and dependent parts. The weight will increase and the blood pressure rise, possibly to levels causing encephalopathy. Drowsiness and vomiting are common and bleeding may be troublesome — especially in the haemolytic uraemic syndrome.

Treatment

General

The usual plan should be followed:
1 Weigh and measure.
2 Assessment of hydration.
3 Blood pressure measured.
4 Blood for haemoglobulin, electrolytes, creatinine, acid/base studies, calcium, phosphorus and alkaline phosphatase analyses, *plus* any specific blood tests, e.g. serum protein and complement.
5 Urine for urea, creatinine, sodium, osmolality, microscopy and culture analyses.
6 Strict maintenance of fluid balance chart.

Most cases will need access to a vein so an intravenous infusion of 0.18% saline and 4.3% dextrose should be given to supply insensible loss (see pp. 40).

Specific

Prerenal failure: If the history, examination and laboratory evidence suggests this diagnosis then fluid replacement should be given and a diuretic challenge given. The usual agents are frusemide, mannitol or dopamine; frusemide 5 mg/kg is given when fluid replacement is underway and should produce a urine flow of at least 0.1 ml/kg/hour. If this fails it can be repeated but the evidence that regular administration influences the course of ARF is dubious. Sixty ml/m^2 of mannitol 12.5% intravenously should produce a urine output greater than 12 ml/m^2/hour within an hour of administration. The risk is that with intrinsic renal failure this bolus may make extracellular fluid overload worse. This risk should not be undertaken if there are serious doubts about the diagnosis, and should certainly not be repeated if the response is meagre. If frusemide or mannitol succeed then treatment should proceed as for isotonic dehydration (see p. 48), but both may cause sodium to be excreted and this will need to be replaced. Dopamine infusions have been beneficial in adults with prerenal failure; at low doses (2–5 µg/kg/min) renal bloodflow improves and diuresis and natriuresis follow. At rates of 5–15 µg/kg/min cardiac-stimulating effects are added to the renal vasodilatory effects. Above these rates the renal bloodflow falls. Although dopamine may not prevent dialysis being required it may produce a urine output sufficient to avoid fluid overload and allow the administration of energy.

Intrinsic renal failure: If the treatment of prerenal failure with adequate fluid replacement does not improve urine flow and clearance of urea and potassium, or if it is clear from the history that prerenal failure is unlikely, specific treatment for intrinsic renal failure is required. The principle is to maintain the patient at an approximately constant weight without fluid overload, hypertension and pulmonary oedema, to maintain the serum potassium within safe limits, and to provide adequate nutrition.

Fluids: The volume of fluid allowed is that of insensible loss (0.5–1.5 ml/kg/hour depending on age) plus output from kidneys, gastrointestinal tract and venesection. It is helpful to calculate serial 4-hour allowances. This volume includes fluid in food and fluid for tablet taking, and this is a severe restriction in a small child whose accustomed source of comfort is a drink. The fluid allowance should be used to provide as much energy as possible. If the fluid limits are exceeded the weight and blood pressure will rise and dialysis will be required. If nutrition is inadequate then tissue breakdown may lead to a reduction in dry body weight. If the measured body weight is not falling then fluid will have been retained, again making dialysis necessary.

Electrolytes: Maintenance allowances of sodium and chloride are given and any deficit or continuing loss replenished. Potassium is not given unless dialysis is being undertaken.

In hyperkalaemia, if the serum potassium rises above 8.0 mmol/l fatal cardiac arrhythmias may occur. The methods used for reducing the level are given on p. 61. A low potassium diet should be used from the start of renal failure; if diet and resin therapy do not control the serum potassium then dialysis is required.

Nutrition: As in any other fluid and electrolyte derangement a short-lived period of malnutrition lasting 48–72 hours can be ignored — especially in a previously healthy child. If the conditions persist longer then it is more likely that malnutrition will, in itself, influence the outcome. Studies in adults have shown that the survival of patients who were well supplied with nutrition was better than for those who were not.

Plans for nutrition should be made early in the management. A target daily intake of dietary constituents (energy, protein, fat and carbohydrate) should be agreed with the help of a dietitian, though allowing the child to eat as much of his or her normal food as possible will probably help morale. Account must be taken of the sodium, potassium, calcium and phosphate content and the amount of fluid allowed, and calorie supplements may be required. A decision also needs to be made about the route of feeding.

If the oral intake by day is inadequate then a fine-bore nasogastric tube might be passed and the calories topped up overnight towards the target level using milk or a proprietary calorie source. Care must be taken not to cause diarrhoea due to the hypertonic feed attracting water into the gut; volumes may therefore need to be reduced. If the child is vomiting, or for some other reason the enteral route is unavailable, then intravenous nutrition must be given (see Chapter 11). In the sick child who is having peritoneal dialysis and intravenous feeding, hyperglycaemia may be troublesome and require insulin therapy; one sign of improving nutrition may be a fall in insulin requirement.

One result of pursuing an active nutritional policy is that dialysis is more likely to be required. This is not to be condemned since the techniques now available are able to give efficient dialysis treatment and keep the child in a good general condition, and complications such as infection are less likely to develop than when starvation was practised.

Dialysis: This may be done through the peritoneum or by haemodialysis. In children, the large surface area of the peritoneum makes dialysis more efficient and is the preferred route in the younger child. Older children may find the restraint and continual dialysis process demoralizing, and in young adults with disorders causing massive tissue breakdown peritoneal dialysis may not control the metabolic deficit. In these circumstances haemodialysis may be preferred. Percutaneous catheters may be inserted into large veins (femoral or subclavian) making arteriovenous shunt surgery unnecessary.

1 *Peritoneal dialysis (PD)*. This technique is straightforward to describe but sometimes presents difficulties even in a renal unit, and should not be embarked upon lightly or without some experience.

The child is sedated (with care because of the effect of compromised renal function on drug excretion) and a small area one-third of the way down a line from umbilicus to symphysis pubis is infiltrated with local anaesthetic (lignocaine 1%). An intravenous catheter is inserted into the peritoneal cavity and 30 ml/kg of dialysate fluid run in to provide some abdominal distension. The catheter is withdrawn and replaced by a larger catheter inserted (with some force) with the aid of a trocar. More fluid (about 50 ml/kg) is run in to create a large reservoir which is repeatedly drained and replenished. When metabolic equilibrium is restored the catheter can be removed and a new one inserted for subsequent dialysis; otherwise overnight or daytime regular PD may be done if return of renal function is delayed.

The main disadvantage of PD is infection; the risk of peritonitis will be reduced by minimal tampering with the dialysate fluid bags and an automatic PD machine will be useful here. Various dialysis fluids are available, the fluid in general use being slightly hypertonic with a Na^+ concentration of 140 mmol/l. Water and electrolyte removal can be achieved using very hypertonic glucose solutions, but care must be taken in case dehydration and collapse occur. The dialysate fluids contains no potassium and this will have to be added when the plasma level falls to below 4 mmol/l.

2 *Haemodialysis (HD)*. Although appearing more formidable than PD, haemodialysis has the advantage of a short duration of treatment and less nursing time being required. The major drawback is achieving and maintaining access to the circulation, but percutaneous catheters have made this more straightforward and therapy, such as plasma exchange, may also be given. Haemodialysis may be done daily for 2-3 hours with adequate

biochemical control, and a calculated amount of water is removed to be replaced with energy-containing fluid over the next 24 hours. In protracted ARF the frequency of dialysis may be reduced and can by done from home as an outpatient procedure.

Haemofiltration: Haemofiltration has recently been developed for ARF, particularly in adults, but there is no reason why children should not be similarly treated. In this technique blood is removed from the body and passed through a cartridge containing special membranes which allow the passage of an ultrafiltrate of plasma. Very large volumes of ECF can be removed by this method and adequate space left for nutrition. Dialysis will be required for removal of nitrogenous waste and potassium — but less frequently than when the patient is managed by haemodialysis alone.

Chronic renal failure

Children who are uraemic may behave like diabetics with a fixed urine output driven by the osmotic load of urea. Some of these patients will have a primary renal condition which causes salt wasting. These patients must not have fluids withheld pre-operatively or renal function will be further compromised and symptomatic uraemia may supervene. Fluid should therefore be given intravenously and the infusion started as soon as there is any restriction on oral intake. Maintenance fluid volumes should be given as 0.45% saline/2.5% dextrose, and any abnormal losses corrected. Sometimes the obligatory urine output exceeds that supplied by the renal component of standard maintenance volumes (about 50% of the total maintenance volume) and extra will be required (see Table 8.3). The child's weight and blood pressure should be observed frequently in case fluid overload or depletion

Table 8.3 Maintenance fluid required during chronic renal failure (CRF), using as an example a 9.6 kg child with CRF undergoing surgery

Maintenance volume = 100 ml/kg/24 hours	= 960 ml
	= 40 ml/hour
Expected urine output ≃ 48 ml/kg/24 hours	≃ 20 ml/hour
but if observed urine output = 30 ml/hour then total fluid volume for next hour is *50 ml*	

occur. Plasma urea and electrolytes should be measured daily, and hourly urine volumes recorded. This is best done without using a bladder catheter but if there is any doubt about collection then the risks should be accepted and the bladder catheterized.

If salt depletion occurs as, for instance, in an intercurrent illness, then the estimated deficits should be replaced as isotonic saline with sodium bicarbonate supplements if there is a severe acidosis. Maintenance volumes and fluids (plus a supplement for high urine volumes if necessary) may then be given.

Children on dialysis undergoing surgery usually cannot have liberal fluids. The principle is to assess the average daily urine output and add an allowance for insensible loss. This total is the maximum allowed over 24 hours, and can be supplied as 0.18% saline in 5% dextrose. Abnormal losses can, of course, be replaced volume for volume and electrolytes mmol for mmol (though it is usually best to avoid giving potassium). If the maximum allowance is exceeded then the risk of volume overload becomes greater, bringing the need for emergency dialysis and heparinization (if haemodialysis is being used) in the recently operated patient.

9

Poisoning

Although many children are admitted to hospital because of accidental poisoning the vast majority suffer no ill effects and very few (about 20 per year in the UK) die. A substantial number require routine observation or supportive treatment; these are children who are poisoned with drugs such as tricyclic antidepressants (now the commonest cause of death), paracetamol, salicylates and opiates.

General principles

The poison should be identified, the amount taken estimated (if in doubt, it is safer to overestimate), and the time since ingestion calculated. Blood, urine and vomit should be saved for analysis. The stomach should be emptied by inducing emesis with ipecacuanha paediatric emetic mixture, 14 mg (10 ml) for children aged 6–18 months and 21 mg (15 ml) for children of 18 months or more, followed by generous liquids. This should not be given if petroleum or corrosive poisons have been taken. The dose of ipecacuanha may be repeated if vomiting does not occur within 20 minutes. It is not worth causing emesis if the drug has been ingested more than 4 hours, except in poisoning from tricyclic antidepressants and opiates (up to 8 hours) and salicylates (up to 24 hours) where gastric emptying may be delayed. If the child is stuporose (or worse) gastric lavage should be done with a secure airway rather than risking aspiration of vomit into the lungs.

Respiration and blood pressure should be measured and maintained by mechanical or pharmacological support if necessary. Maintenance fluids should be given and deficits and abnormal losses replaced. Convulsions should be stopped and prevented by anticonvulsants such as diazepam, phenytoin or phenobarbitone.

Tricyclic antidepressants

These are usually prescribed for adult mental illness or childhood enuresis but their lethal potential is often underestimated by doctors and laymen. The effects are usually of central stimulation with confusion, irritability, extrapyramidal rigidity and jerking followed by convulsions and coma. Cardiovascular effects are tachycardia, ventricular ectopic beats and conduction defects.

Treatment

1 Activated charcoal 1 g/kg should be given *after* the emesis from ipecacuanha, providing no more than 3 hours have elapsed since the ingestion.
2 Forced diuresis, dialysis and haemoperfusion are not helpful.
3 Convulsions or extreme irritability should be treated with diazepam.
4 Cardiotoxicity: beta blockade will reduce tachycardia, and lignocaine may suppress ventricular ectopic beats. Conduction defects are rare but may require a pacemaker.
5 Hypotension: dopamine infusion 1 µg/kg/minute and increased according to response.
6 Maintenance fluid volumes may have to be increased by 5% to allow for extra loss in convulsive or other catabolic states.
7 Cardiac arrest: spectacular recoveries have been documented after long periods of cardiac standstill supported by external cardiac massage.
8 Patients with refractory cardiac tachyarrhythmias or neurological symptoms could be given physostigmine 0.5 mg intravenously over 2 minutes and repeated if necessary. Further doses may be required at 2–4 hours. This therapy is controversial and hazardous as it causes bradycardia and asystole.

Paracetamol

Deaths have been recorded with the ingestion of as little as 10 g of paracetamol. The drug is hepatotoxic and liver damage becomes clinically apparent 3–4 days after ingestion. An early sign of liver toxicity is prolongation of the prothrombin time. Other toxic effects of paracetamol are on the heart, kidneys and brain. Despite its wide use as an antipyretic severe paracetamol poisoning is rare in childhood. Blood should be taken to assess the paracetamol level when the child is first seen, and if there is any possibility that a toxic dose has been ingested specific treatment should begin immediately. If therapy is delayed beyond 10 hours it will be ineffective, whereas therapy can easily be discontinued if the paracetamol level is unexpectedly low. Figure 9.1 shows the toxicity of paracetamol related to plasma levels.

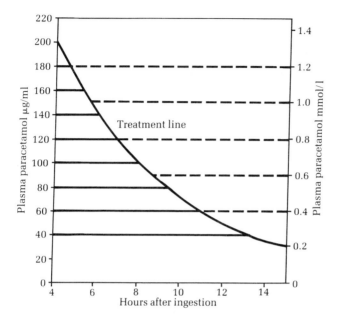

Figure 9.1 Plasma paracetamol concentrations in relation to time after overdosage as a guide to prognosis. Treatment is indicated in patients with values just below or above the treatment line. From Prescott, L.F., 1978, *Health Bulletin* **4,** 204.

Treatment

1 Emesis.

2 Charcoal.

3 Support circulation and respiration — but coma is extremely rare unless a massive dose taken.

4 Maintenance fluids.

5 Specific treatment (*must start before 10 hours*): acetylcysteine 150 mg/kg given intravenously and immediately, followed by acetylcysteine diluted in 5% dextrose 12.5 mg/kg/hour for 4 hours and then 5 mg/kg/hour for 15 hours; or methionine 30 mg/kg orally every 4 hours × 4 doses.

Salicylates

Overdosage of salicylates results in poisoning of a number of major body systems causing respiratory stimulation and alkalosis, metabolic acidosis (more likely in a young child), hypoglycaemia and hypoprothrombinaemia. There is a generalized increase in the metabolic rate with hyperpyrexia and sweating. Dehydration and excessive renal sodium and potassium loss are common. Blood should be taken to obtain a salicylate level, and the severity of intoxication assessed using the nomogram in Figure 9.2. Ingestion of more than 300 mg/kg is usually followed by severe symptoms.

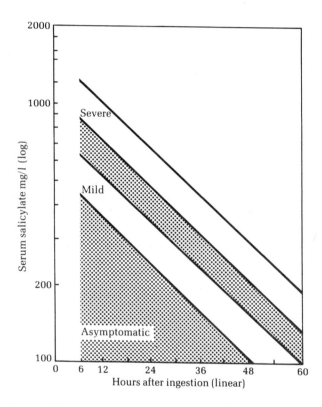

Figure 9.2 The relation between the measured serum salicylate and the time after ingestion of the drug that the salicylate level was obtained for with the anticipated clinical severity of the intoxication. From Done, A.K. 1960, *Pediatrics* **26**, 800.

Treatment

1 Emesis.
2 Charcoal.
3 Support circulation and respiration (in severe poisoning).
4 Maintenance fluids plus 5% to allow for increased metabolic rate in mild poisoning. Sodium requirements may be greater than usual. Losses from vomit, sweating, etc. should be replaced.
5 Vitamin K 2.5 mg given intravenously.
6 Measurement and correction of acid/base status (usually acidosis) 4–6 hourly: this carries serious risks (see p. 78) and bicarbonate should only be given if the pH is less than 7.1. Very small quantities (1–2 mmol/kg) of dilute bicarbonate should be used.
7 Measurement of blood glucose every 4 hours.

Forced alkaline diuresis works by decreasing the time that a drug is in the renal tubule and therefore likely to be reabsorbed, and by increasing the ionized component of the drug to promote excretion. Weakly acidic drugs like aspirin will be more ionized in an alkaline environment. Forced alkaline diuresis was widely used in the treatment of salicylate poisoning, but complications such as fluid overload, hypokalaemia and severe acid/base derangement may occur. Two specific indications are blood levels which suggest that moderate or severe poisoning will occur and the development of convulsions and coma with severe hyperpnoea. A regimen for forced alkaline diuresis is shown in Table 9.1, but in paediatric practice measures 4–6 above are most commonly employed and preferred. When there is major poisoning (salicylate level approaching 2000 mg/l), severe acidosis or renal failure, dialysis (haemodialysis or peritoneal) will remove the drug effectively with a lesser risk of metabolic catastrophe.

Opiates

Lomotil (diphenoxylate and atropine) and Distalgesic (dextropropoxyphene with paracetamol) contain sufficient opiate to cause respiratory depression in children. The specific reversing agent is naloxone 5 mg/kg intramuscularly or intravenously and this may need to be repeated in severe poisoning. Maintenance fluids should be given. Persisting symptoms or later appearance of toxicity may be caused by the other drug in combination.

Table 9.1 Forced alkaline diuresis

Diuresis
1.5–2 × maintenance volumes: urine output 2–4 ml/kg/hour, urine specific gravity<1010

The diuresis may be promoted by diuretics such as:
1 mannitol (osmotic) 1 g/kg over 20 minutes, once only
2 frusemide 1 mg/kg; may be repeated if urine output falls and if clinical and biochemical progress is favourable

Note:
1 diuretics should not be given until dehydration is corrected or there is a risk of inducing renal failure
2 The maintenance fluid should contain: (i) dextrose as hypoglycaemia is likely; (ii) Na 30–60 mmol/l; 0.18% saline/4.3% dextrose can be used at first but 0.45% saline/2.5% dextrose may be required if sodium losses are great. The dextrose concentration may be insufficient to maintain blood glucose; and (iii) when urine output is established add KCl 20 mmol/l but be prepared to increase this

Forced diuresis may be sufficient on its own but if there is a metabolic acidosis with a compromised circulation, sodium bicarbonate may be given

Alkali (if blood pH 7.1)
$NaHCO_3$ 1–2 mmol/kg intravenously over 1 hour followed by 0.5 mmol/kg 3-hourly. This should be varied according to blood acid/base balance and urine pH (which rarely gets to 8) taken before each dose of bicarbonate. If the acid/base status is improving then the bicarbonate should be withheld. When the serum salicylate is consistently falling alkali should be discontinued and the infusion rate decreased

Note that alkali therapy predisposes to hypokalaemia

Other poisons, bites and stings

Barbiturates, iron and domestic cleansers may all be ingested by children. Maintenance fluids plus restoration of deficit or abnormal loss should be given. Substantial amounts of fluid, electrolyte or H^+ may be lost if there is profuse diarrhoea or vomiting, especially if induced by purging.

Snake and insect bites may cause considerable soft tissue swelling and sequestration of fluid from the ECF. In snake bites this will be exacerbated by the vomiting and diarrhoea. Although direct renal damage from venom is described it is much more likely that renal functional impairment will be caused by hypovolaemia and will improve with restoration of the circulation. Antivenoms are seldom needed in the UK.

10

Other Metabolic Conditions

Adrenocortical failure

An acute Addisonian crisis may occur in the older child during withdrawal of suppressive corticosteroid therapy, or rarely because of maldevelopment, cancer (and surgery), tuberculous destruction or auto-immune Addison's disease. The most common cause of acute adrenal failure is in infants with congenital adrenal hyperplasia resulting from a recessively inherited deficit of adrenal 21-hydroxylase enzyme. Two-thirds of these babies have a salt-losing form of this enzyme which usually presents during the first month of life. The condition may be recognized in a masculinized female at birth, but otherwise the infant thrives for a week or so and then rapidly deteriorates with vomiting, jaundice, diarrhoea and circulatory collapse. The symptoms are not specific and could be caused by any life-threatening illness in the neonatal period. Figure 10.1 shows the biochemical lesion. It should be remembered that any child taking corticosteroid tablets or those who have adrenocortical insufficiency from any cause, develop an acute crisis in an intercurrent illness or during surgery.

Effects

Aldosterone is a potent mineralocorticoid which promotes sodium reabsorption in the distal tubule of the kidney — exchanging it for potassium or hydrogen ion. Hydrocortisone also has some mineralocorticoid properties, and cortisol precursors may competitively inhibit aldosterone action on the distal tubule. Absence of these hormones means that:

1 Sodium and chloride are lost in the urine.
2 Water is lost with the sodium, causing polyuria.
3 The plasma sodium falls.
4 Potassium and H^+ are retained; this is exacerbated by the hypovolaemia due to sodium and water loss and the consequent fall in glomerular filtration.

Absence of hydrocortisone leads to deranged protein and carbohydrate metabolism with:

5 Hypoglycaemia.

Diagnosis

The condition should be considered by any doctor dealing with an

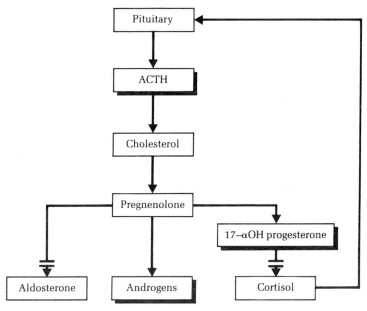

$\perp$ = site of enzyme deficit.

Results: **1** Impaired production of:
(a) aldosterone → salt-losing state.
(b) cortisol → tendency to hypoglycaemia and/or hypothermia.
2 Excessive production of:
(a) androgen. In boys → larger penis and smaller testes than usual in infants. In girls → masculinization.
(b) ACTH (adrenocorticotrophic hormone) → production of aldosterone/cortisol precursors (e.g. 17–αOH progesterone) and androgens.

Figure 10.1 The effects of 21-hydroxylase deficiency in congenital adrenal hyperplasia.

acutely ill infant. A clue may be that the baby is very much more ill than would be expected from the history. The genitalia need careful examination.

   Investigations may show:

1 A low plasma sodium.

2 An inappropriately high urine sodium or chloride (in the face of hyponatraemia the infant kidney should be able to shut off sodium excretion; in hypovolaemic collapse from other conditions such as septicaemia there should be negligible sodium in the urine).

3 Hyperkalaemia, possibly with ECG changes.

4 Hypoglycaemia.

Additionally blood should be taken in order to examine the 17-α OH-progesterone level, and chromosomes (a buccal smear may be done in an emergency). A 24-hour urine sample should be taken to calculate hourly volume measurements, and steroid and pregnanetriol levels.

Treatment

Provide warmth and, perhaps, oxygen.

1 Fluid loss: 0.9% saline and 5% dextrose 20 ml/kg over 30 minutes then 0.9% saline and 5% dextrose in maintenance amounts, but aim to give 60% of the 24-hour volume in the first 8 hours (this is because the action of adrenal hormone replacement will be to replenish the ECF and overhydration is a risk). The position should be reviewed every 4 hours. When the plasma Na^+ reaches 132 mmol/l change maintenance to 0.18% saline/4.3% dextrose. When oral feeds start then sodium chloride supplement will be needed — starting with 100 mg/kg/24 hours in divided doses with feeds.

2 Hyperkalaemia: treat as shown on p. 61 but insulin should not be given.

3 Hypoglycaemia: dextrose 5% is included in the rehydrating fluid. If hypoglycaemia is refractory use 10 ml of 50% infusion diluted with water.

4 Steroid replacement:

(a) Glucocorticoid: hydrocortisone 2 mg/kg intravenously for acute replacement; a further dose of 1 mg/kg should be given at 4 and 8 hours. Replacement therapy with cortisone acetate 2 mg/kg daily should be started at the same time but when the baby's condition is stable and oral fluids are taken then replacement therapy using the physician's preferred glucocorticoid can be started (e.g. hydrocortisone 16 mg/m² a.m. and 8 mg/m² p.m.).

(b) Mineralocorticoid: immediate treatment with deoxycortone pivalate 25 mg intramuscularly. This may need to be repeated within the next 24 hours; a further dose should be given on the second day. When oral feeds start add fludrocortisone 5 µg/kg/24 hours by mouth.

During the treatment the parents should be told the diagnosis and its implications for assignment of sex, growth and future surgery.

Surgery

Like the diabetic child, a patient with adrenal failure will need careful management:

1 Give cortisone acetate 2 mg/kg 12 hours pre-operatively and 1 mg/kg with premedication; then 1 mg/kg/24 hours postoperatively until oral steroids are tolerated.

2 Give hydrocortisone 50 mg intravenously with induction of anaesthesia and 3-hourly thereafter *during the operation.*

3 Mineralocorticoid: use deoxycortone pivalate daily until oral medication is resumed.

4 Fluids: 0.9% saline/5% dextrose maintenance pre-operatively, then 0.45% saline/5% dextrose thereafter.

The doses of glucocorticoids and fluids may need to be modified if the clinical course dictates it.

Inborn errors of metabolism

Vomiting and rapid sighing respiration from metabolic acidosis may be the presenting feature of an inborn error of amino acid or other organic acid metabolism. The differential diagnosis of metabolic acidosis is shown in Table 10.1. The amino-acidopathies present during the first month of life with non-specific symptoms such as vomiting, which may progress to a life-threatening illness with collapse. Some of these children are mistakenly diagnosed as having some surgical condition, such as pyloric stenosis. Definitive treatment is by regulating dietary amino acid intake (in propionic acidaemia) or vitamin B_{12} therapy (for some forms of methylmalonic acidaemia). The acute treatment is to make good the deficits produced by vomiting and to give maintenance fluids. Sodium bicarbonate may need to be given to combat the acidosis. In cases of extreme acid/base and electrolyte abnormality (particularly with raised blood ammonia levels) peritoneal dialysis may be helpful.

Table 10.1 Differential diagnosis of severe metabolic acidosis in children

Carbohydrate metabolism
    diabetes mellitus
    glycogen storage disease
Organic acid metabolism, including:
    methylmalonic acidaemia
    propionic acidaemia
    isovaleric acidaemia
Endocrine disease
    congenital adrenal hyperplasia
Renal disease
    renal tubular acidosis
    renal failure
Poisoning
    aspirin

SIADH — water retention syndromes

Antidiuretic hormone is secreted from the posterior pituitary gland in response to such conditions as hypovolaemia, plasma hyperosmolality and stimulation of carotid receptors. Its effect is on the distal renal tubule and collecting duct, making them permeable to water, and thus it is a conserving hormone. In some pathological states such as chest disease, head injuries, intracranial disease and overwhelming septicaemic illness, ADH is released in the absence of hypertonicity or hypovolaemia and with normal kidney and adrenal function. Such hormone production forms part of the syndrome of inappropriate antidiuretic hormone secretion (SIADH).

The hallmarks are:

1 Clinical: gradual neurological deterioration (plasma Na^+ < 125 mmol/l) progressing to stupor, coma and fits (plasma Na^+ < 115 mmol/l).

2 Biochemical: plasma Na^+ and osmolality are low; and urine Na^+ and osmolality are high — inappropriately so, considering the plasma levels.

Treatment

Treatment is by fluid restriction. Intake should be reduced to 75% maintenance; further reductions to 50% or even 30% maintenance volumes are sometimes required. If the plasma Na $^+$ remains low or convulsions occur then the infusion of hypertonic saline is justified: 3% sodium chloride 3 mmol/kg (or 6 ml/kg) — half over 30 minutes and the rest over 3 hours.

Hypercalcaemia

Most commonly the result of excessive treatment with vitamin D preparations, hypercalcaemia is still a rare disorder in children. Table 10.2 summarizes the causes.

Table 10.2   Causes of hypercalcaemia

Hyperparathyroidism (primary or secondary, usually in renal failure)
Idiopathic hypercalcaemia of infancy
Vitamin D intoxication
Familial benign hypercalcaemia
Leukaemia and other malignancies
Immobilization
Sarcoidosis

Diagnosis

This may be obvious from the history, especially in a patient taking vitamin D; symptoms being anorexia, vomiting, constipation and abdominal pain, polyuria and thirst resulting from loss of the concentrating power of the kidney. Failure to thrive is a common symptom in infancy. The condition may be asymptomatic — coming to light in a biochemistry profile. The serum calcium will be raised above 2.75 mmol/l but may be as high as 4 mmol/l. The phosphate level in the blood will depend on the primary disease — in hyperparathyroidism it is low but in renal insufficiency it will be high. When the phosphate is high and the calcium × phosphate solubility product exceeds five, symptoms of metastatic calcification (red, itchy eyes and generlized pruritis) may occur.

Treatment

The primary disorder may need specific attention, withdrawal of vitamin D, parathyroidectomy, dietary restriction, etc.

1 Fluids. Patients may be considerably dehydrated and a brisk diuresis may reduce the serum calcium to safe levels. Deficit should be replaced with isotonic saline: maintenance fluid should be 0.45% saline/2.5% dextrose and, when urine is voided, potassium chloride 20 mmol/l (or sometimes more) should be added. The sodium content may need to be varied depending on natriuresis; if in doubt 6-hourly urine specimens should have the electrolyte content measured and the output replaced intravenously.

2 Diuretics. Frusemide 1 mg/kg 6-hourly when dehydration has been corrected. This is calciuric as well as natriuretic. When the calcium is below 3 mmol/l treatment may be discontinued.

3 Steroids. Prednisolone 2 mg/kg/24 hours will help reduce the serum calcium within a week or so — except in hyperparathyroidism.

4 Phosphate. Providing the serum potassium is not high oral phosphate 1–2 g/day will reduce the serum calcium.

5 Calcitonin. This acts by blocking the movement of calcium out of bone and into the blood. Five units/kg are given twice daily at the same time as starting steroid therapy.

6 Mithramycin. This antibiotic, which inhibits RNA synthesis, is used to control hypercalcaemia in malignant disease.

7 Dialysis. Patients with renal failure who cannot tolerate intravenous fluids, or who cannot produce a diuresis, may benefit from a period of dialysis while the serum calcium is reduced. It is possible that when this is controlled dialysis may not be required.

Induction of remissions in malignant disease

Most children presenting with malignant disease, including leukaemia, will have at least 1 kg of abnormal tissue (10^{12} cells). In most cases extremely rapid breakdown of this tissue begins within hours of starting treatment, and the patient is at grave risk from the biochemical sequelae. Cell lysis allows sudden release of potassium, phosphate and uric acid, nephropathy may occur from the huge filtered load of urates and other metabolites, whilst the hyperkalaemia and hypocalcaemia may reach dangerous levels. Renal excretion is encouraged by:

1 Intravenous fluids at twice the usual maintenance rate.

2 Allopurinol 300 mg/m²/24 hours.

3 Alkalinization with $NaHCO_3$ 3 mmol/kg/24 hours adjusted as necessary to keep urine pH > 7. Intravenous fluids should therefore be given as 5% dextrose since the added $NaHCO_3$ will give adequate amounts of sodium.

4 Acetezolamide may also be used as an alkaninizing agent. The adult dose is 500 mg q.d.s., and dosage for children is 250 mg b.d.–t.d.s. If possible all the above should be given 24 hours before cytotoxic therapy is started.

Plasma levels of sodium, potassium, chloride, calcium, phosphate and uric acid should be measured daily during the first few days of therapy until a safe, stable state has been reached.

11

Nutrition

In recent years the importance of adequate nutrition in the ill or convalescent patient has become emphasized. For short illnesses or surgery, near starvation lasting 48–72 hours is acceptable in the child who was previously well nourished. If this period of malnutrition is prolonged then morbidity will be greater; weight loss will occur, wound healing may be delayed, and infection may be more likely. In the past, procrastination about feeding occurred, in the hope that the clinical condition would improve and allow oral intake to be absorbed. This is now unacceptable; in certain conditions, such as neonatal surgery, care of the newborn child with very low birth weight, renal failure and the treatment of some malignant diseases, failure of oral nutriton can be predicted and intravenous feeding should be started immediately. When food intolerance follows some gastrointestinal condition or where there is inflammatory bowel disease or other prolonged illness then weight loss, progressive anaemia and lowering of plasma protein levels should not be tolerated. The nutritional requirements of the sick child will be up to 50% greater than the healthy child. Unfortunately the sick child may be anorexic, nauseated, demoralized and have no peripheral veins. This should be a challenge and not a reason for despair.

Access

The routes available for nutrition are enteral, by mouth or nasogastric or nasojejunal tube, or parenteral via intravenous cannula. The latter may be peripheral, requiring frequent changes of site and the risk of exhausting all available veins; central lines are placed in the vena cava from the internal jugular, subclavian or other peripheral veins. Their major hazard is the introduction of infection to the sick patient, and once a septicaemia occurs the line usually has to be removed. Opinions differ about who should place them, and where. There is considerable support for their placement in the operating theatre as an aseptic surgical procedure.

Enteral feeding

Here we assume that the child cannot (or will not) consume sufficient nutrients from a normal diet for their age. If the child is not vomiting or there is no other impediment to absorption of nutrients then the enteral route is preferred, and intravenous nutrition avoided since it is complicated and costly. Clinical conditions where this would be required are head injuries, inflammatory bowel disease and acute renal failure.

If the gut is to be used for some time a fine-bore silastic tube should be introduced, sometimes using radiographic control; for short-term feeding a PVC nasogastric tube will suffice. Most patients will start on clear fluids, water, 5% dextrose or some electrolyte compound. It is important to introduce the enteral feed slowly in case vomiting or osmotic diarrhoea occur (requiring replacement as abnormal loss). One method is to dilute the full strength feed to 25%, 50% and 75% strength over successive days. If intravenous nutrition is already being used it can cover the deficit; when the enteral feed is being absorbed the intravenous route may be abandoned. Enteral tube feeding may be carried out for many weeks and patients have been maintained on it at home.

The major risk — particularly in the infant — is that of regurgitation of feed and inhalation. Nurses should watch for choking, coughing or increased abdominal distension. This complication can be avoided if small volumes are used at first and if the flow rate is controlled by an infusion pump. Use of hospital-prepared solutions through fine-bore tubes has been criticized because of bacterial contamination and tube blockage causing difficulties in infusion.

There are now many proprietary nutritionally-complete formulae allowing greater flexibility for use with differing clinical circumstances. Skilled paediatric dietetic help is invaluable in making the correct choice of diet. Such long-term enteral feeding needs some experience in its management; it is expensive and the aims of using it should be clear. Success must not only be judged on changes in body weight; but a detailed discussion of nutritional physiology is beyond the scope of this book.

Parenteral feeding

This requires the services of many disciplines, including medical, surgical, laboratory, pharmacy and dietetic personnel, and best results will be obtained by those who have some experience of the technique. Three decisions need to be made:

1 When to start treatment: at the start of predictable clinical circumstances, for example acute renal failure, or when enteral nutrition fails for more than a few days in a patient who is not recovering rapidly.

2 Venous access: central or peripheral.

3 Regimen to use: many different schemes have been devised. All are based on recommended daily intakes, but the solutions used to provide this energy vary.

(a) *Carbohydrate:* hypertonic glucose solutions are used almost exclusively. When central lines are used there is less risk of venous thrombosis; hypertonic glucose solutions rapidly thrombose peripheral veins. The other complication is of hyperosmolar dehydration if the glucose is not metabolized efficiently; an osmotic diuresis may occur and insulin therapy be necessary.

(b) *Fat:* an excellent source of energy. Fat emulsions of various strengths are available and may have to provide the principal energy source when peripheral veins are used. They are not recommended in the septic patient or those with liver disease or thrombocytopenia, and there is anxiety about the accumulation of fat in the tissues of very small infants. If fat solutions are not used then carbohydrate will be the main energy source. Allergic reactions, haematological abnormalities and jaundice may complicate fat infusions.

(c) *Protein:* nitrogen sources are presented as protein hydrolysates or crystaline amino acid solutions. The concentrations of amino acids vary and some solutions contain glucose. The risks of protein infusion are small and mainly result in amino acid imbalance, with elevated levels in the newborn, and in metabolic acidosis and liver dysfunction with raised ammonia and transaminase levels.

Technique

The nutritional line should not be used for blood sampling or any other infusions (drugs, blood, etc.). The more the line is tampered with, the greater the risk of infection; the sepsis rate is inversely proportional to the skill and experience of the team. The risk of infection is reduced by using a multipore filter in the circuit of the dextrose/amino acid infusion; by changing bottles, giving sets, connections and filters daily using an aseptic technique; and by changing the site of peripheral infusions as soon as there is reddening, swelling or a reduction of infusion volume not accounted for by changes in position of the intravenous cannula.

The infusion should be controlled by a pump but this needs careful nursing observation since extravasation of fluid may cause serious skin damage. Frequent blood cultures must be taken and clinical signs of infection watched for. These include unstable body temperature (high or low), rashes, reduced clearance of lipid and hyperglycaemia. The site of entry of the catheter and the exit of any tunnelled central line should be protected by daily cleansing with antiseptic and by covering with a sterile occlusive dressing. Some teams use creams impregnated with antibacterial or antifungal agents.

Antibiotics should not be given prophylactically during parenteral feeding but should be commenced at the first sign of trouble. Intralipid should not be used when there is systemic sepsis; however energy provisions should not be reduced in case the patient's ability to overcome the infection is prejudiced.

Intravenous infusion regimen

The regimen given below (p. 110) has been used in infants in the Bristol neonatal intensive care units; such regimens vary and there are likely to be local preferences. Allowance is made for infants whose birth weight is less than 1500 g because they may not tolerate even 10% dextrose without developing hyperglycaemia. A glycosuric osmotic diuresis and more dilute solutions are sometimes used. Fluid volumes are gradually increased over the first week of life as shown in Table 11.1. Small-for-gestational-age infants may start at one day ahead; these infants tolerate intralipid particularly poorly. Table 11.2 shows a modification of the infant regimen suitable for children up to puberty.

These two schedules use three basic solutions: (1) dextrose (which may be given at various concentrations, e.g. 10%, 20% or 25%); (2) vamin-dextrose; and (3) intralipid. All have some additions to the bottle and these should be prepared in the pharmacy under aseptic conditions. It is preferable to introduce parenteral feeding gradually: 3–5 days are usually required. One regimen uses maintenance solutions to provide 75%, 50% and 25% of fluid volume so that by day 4 total parenteral nutrition is being given.

Table 11.1 Bristol hospitals' intravenous feeding schedule for newborn infants > 1500 g (figures in brackets = < 1500 g)

Age	Infusion solutions (ml/kg/24 hours)						
	10% dextrose	10% dextrose electrolytes (day 2 only)	Solution 1, 10% dextrose mixture	Solution 2, vamin-dextrose mixture	Solution 3, intralipid mixture	Water for injection or 5% dextrose*	Total volume/kg/ 24 hours
Day 1	60(80)						60(80)
Day 2		90(100–120)					90(100–120)
Day 3			90(110–120)	20(20)			110(130–140)
Day 4			100(120–130)	30(30)			130(150–160)
Day 5			100–110(120–140)	40(40)			140–150(160–180)
Day 6			100–120(120–140)	40(40)	0–10(0–10)†	(0–20)	140–160(160–180)
Day 7			100–120(120–140)	40(40)	0–20(0–20)	(0–20)	140–170(160–180)
Day 8			100–140(120–140)	40(40)	0–20(0–20)	(0–20)	140–180(160–180)
Day 9			100–140(120–140)	40(40)	0–20(0–20)	(0–20)	140–180(160–180)

*Part of solution no. 1 may be replaced by water or 5% dextrose if the infant is hyperglycaemic (blood sugar > 7 mmol/l). If there is glycosuria > 0.5% on clinical testing then use solution no. 1 made up with 5% dextrose.

† Do not start intralipid if bilirubin > 100 µmol/l, or if sepsis is present, or if platelets < 50 000. Initially monitor lipid levels daily, and increase intake as tolerated to maximum of 20 ml/kg/24 hours of 20% intralipid. Start with dose of 10 ml/kg/24 hours 10% intralipid. *Infants under phototherapy:* give an *extra* 1 ml/kg/hour added to burette-water for injection or 5% dextrose. *Infants > 5 days-old and starting intravenous feeding:* start at day 5 on schedule, but do not add intralipid until sepsis is excluded (i.e. 48 hours after cultures are sent). *Small-for-dates infants:* start on schedule at 1 day more than actual age. Check lipid tolerance very carefully as tolerance may be poor.

Table 11.2 Feeding schedules for children aged 7–10 years

Volume of infusion fluid (ml/kg/24 hours)		
Solution 1	(20% dextrose mixture)	30
Solution 2	(vamin-dextrose mixture)	27
Solution 3	(intralipid mixture)	13

For example, for a 30 kg child this volume provides:
2100 ml fluid ($\simeq$ 70 ml/kg)
8400 J energy ($\simeq$ 280 J/kg)
252 g CHO ($\simeq$ 8 g/kg)
80 g fat ($\simeq$ 2.6 g/kg)
50 g protein (amino acids) ($\simeq$ 1.6 g/kg)

Solution 1 (dextrose mixture):
Infant:
500 ml 10% dextrose
2.5 ml Solvito solution (containing vitamins B and C and folic acid)
1 ml 30% sodium chloride solution
2.5 ml concentrated potassium/phosphate solution.
This solution is degenerated by light and the bag and bottle should be protected.
Child:
500 ml 25% dextrose.

Solution 2 (vamin-dextrose mixture):
90 ml vamin-glucose
10 ml Ped-el (calcium, magnesium, iron, zinc, manganese, copper, fluoride, iodide, phosphate, chloride).

Solution 3 (intralipid mixture):
100 ml of 10% or 20% intralipid
5 ml Vitlipid infant vitamin supplement (should be added 1 hour before starting infusion).

Other infusions: To cover surgery, periods of sepsis and the first few days of life of the newborn, other infusion fluids will be required. To provide sufficient energy a hypertonic dextrose solution (e.g. 10%) with added maintenance electrolytes should be used.

Monitoring: These patients need close nursing observation, preferably in a high dependency area. Regular clinical assessment should be made, looking for over- and under-perfusion. Blood pressure, temperature and pulse should be checked 4-hourly. Urine volumes must be recorded and tested for specific gravity (or osmolality) and glucose. Blood glucose (dextrostix, BM-stix) should be measured 8-hourly or more frequently if there is glycosuria, and the child weighed daily.

Blood tests: The following should be tested for *daily* (at first):

Urea, electrolytes, creatinine
pH, bicarbonate
Glucose   Intralipid should have been
Hb, platelets   stopped for 4 hours.
Bilirubin

Lipid content: this is preferably done by nephalometry. An acceptable level is 100 mg/dl. Absence of lipaemia is not sufficient evidence of lipid tolerance although presence of lipid in plasma is evidence of intolerance.

The following should be tested for *twice weekly*:

Calcium
Phosphate
Magnesium
Amino acids
Triglyceride.

The following should be tested for *weekly*:

Transaminases
Alkaline phosphatase
Phosphate
Clotting screen.

Rate of administration: Solutions 1 and 2 are administered together over a 24-hour period; solution 3 over 20 hours allowing 4 hours for blood tests. Hourly target infusion rates must be calculated by medical staff, and progress reviewed regularly. Fluid and energy intake and output charts should be recorded and checked daily.

Weaning from intravenous feeding: The hypertonic solutions cause increased levels of endogenous insulin (and sometimes need exogenous insulin for control). Parenteral nutrition should be gradually discontinued over a 4-day period in a similar way to their institution. When oral nourishment is established the amino acid and lipid infusions may be stopped and decreasing amounts of 10% dextrose infused until blood glucose levels are stable without infusion.

If parenteral nutrition has to stop suddenly then: (1) 6-hourly capillary blood glucose tests must be done; and (2) the period of abstinence should be covered by a 10% dextrose infusion.

Complications:

1 *Metabolic:* metabolic acidosis, trace metal deficiency states, essential fatty acid deficiency.

2 *Hyponatraemia:* if the serum sodium is falling water intake should be reduced or supplemental sodium chloride solution should be given.

3 *Hypernatraemia:* usually represents depletion of ECF water (or excess of solute); give supplemental 5% dextrose.

4 *Hypocalcaemia:* infuse *diluted* calcium gluconate 10% as 0.6 ml/kg/hour of the 10% solution.

5 *Infection:* anticipate and treat. Consider removal of central lines.

6 *Technical:* catheter erosion, brachial plexus injury, surgical emphysema, pneumothorax and many others complicate central line nutrition.

12

Surgery

The scope of paediatric surgery has changed considerably over the last 30 years because of improvements in anaesthetic and surgical technique and in the understanding of temperature control and fluid balance in young patients. Perhaps the most important is the application of knowledge about the response of the adult to surgical stress. In this field, as in many others, it is clear that although there are some broad common principles children behave less like small adults the younger they are. One particular aspect of this is the difference in response to the physical trauma of surgery. Following major surgery or life-threatening illness children experience a much swifter recovery and tolerance of food than would adults in similar circumstances.

Response to surgical stress

Three phases are recognized in the adult and, probably, in children aged 5 years or older: catabolism, early anabolism and late anabolism. It should be realized that these three phases are not clearly defined in children; a 4-month old baby undergoing hernia repair as a day case should be able to take feeds within 12 hours of the procedure and the catabolic phase will be negligible. However an older child with prolonged intra-abdominal sepsis may need several weeks of nutritional support.

Catabolism

This lasts up to one week, and the features are: negative nitrogen and potassium balance, a tendency to sodium and water retention, increased metabolic rate and negative energy balance with a decrease in body weight. These are associated with increased secretion of adrenal cortical and medullary hormones and antidiuretic hormone. The main hazard is that of giving excess parenteral fluids, thus resulting in volume overload and, if excess water is given, hyponatraemia. This period is covered by less than maintenance

114

volumes of glucose and electrolyte solutions, any abnormal loss such as gastric aspiration being replaced volume for volume.

Early anabolism

Early anabolism lasts several weeks. The metabolic rate becomes normal, the body weight will slowly increase and the catabolic process reverses — protein and potassium will be retained for tissue repair and excess sodium and water will be excreted. This transition is crucial and if it is not achieved the patient will deteriorate with poor wound healing and lowered resistance to infection. Energy intake assumes great importance here and should not be jeopardized.

Late anabolism

This a period of restoration of fat stores in adults and children and requires a continuing positive energy balance. In children there is the added aspect of growth; during prolonged periods of surgical (and medical) illness growth will fail because available energy is diverted to meet the increased stress. When this is removed a period of catch-up growth should be anticipated and energy intake must allow for this. It is not uncommon for parents to say that their children have never eaten so well since a particular operation was performed. This may be as much the result of recovery from non-specific surgical stress as from the curative procedure.

Pre-operative management

Elective case

Assuming that the child was previously well nourished and growing adequately then no specific preparation is required. If there has been a prolonged period of ill health which can be medically treated pending a curative operation (e.g. treatment of a chronic urinary tract infection before a urological procedure), then this should be allowed so that catch-up growth can occur with optimal nutrition. In this way the metabolic and nutritional consequences of surgery or its complications may be avoided. Sometimes this breathing space is not available and the risks of the operation are perceptively greater.

Acute case

Here a balance has to be struck between the delay resulting from resuscitation and improvement of the child's general condition, and the risks incurred by delaying surgery. In general, unless there is an immediate threat to life, fluid and electrolyte depletion and acid/base balance should be restored before surgery. To do this the usual plan of deficit restoration, provision of maintenance requirements, and replacement of continuing abnormal losses should be followed for the individual components of water, electrolytes and acid/base balance.

A good example is pyloric stenosis of infancy. These babies are often sodium and water depleted because of vomiting, which will also cause a deficit in potassium and hydrogen ion. The kidneys are unable to reconcile the conflicting claims for conservation of water, sodium, potassium and hydrogen ion, and in these circumstances water and sodium take priority. Sodium is reabsorbed in the distal tubule under the influence of aldosterone, exchanging for potassium and hydrogen ion which are lost in the urine, and the metabolic alkalosis persists.

Treatment is as follows:

1 A nasogastric tube is used and aspirate is replaced hourly, volume for volume, intravenously with a solution of 0.45% saline and potassium chloride 20 mmol/l.

2 Intravenous fluids are given.

(a) Deficit: calculated from body weight and clinical signs. The fluid used is 0.45% saline/4.3% dextrose with KCl 20 mmol/l (if there is severe dehydration give 10 ml/kg 0.9% saline in first hour in addition to restore plasma volume).

(b) Maintenance: 150 ml/kg/24 hours 0.18% saline/4.3% dextrose/KCl 10 mmol/l.

(c) Abnormal losses are covered by **1** above.

Note that the acid/base status does not need specific correction.

The infant should not be operated on until the metabolic deficit is restored. There is no urgency here and no favour is being done to an electrolyte-depleted baby by 'slipping him on to the end of a list'.

Particular attention needs to be given to the child with intestinal obstruction or similar disorders in which copious fluid may be sequestered in the bowel. If this is not vomited, aspirated or passed through the rectum it may not be accounted for in the calculation of the degree of deficit. The amount and composition may be equivalent to an intestinal fistula and if not corrected progressive dehydration may occur. If there is any doubt about replacement volumes then readings from a central venous pressure line will provide guidance.

Peroperative management

Restricted maintenance fluids should be given as in Table 12.1 and abnormal losses corrected. An important loss in a major operation will be blood, and the circulating blood volume of an infant (80 ml/kg) demands that an accurate assessment of loss should be made and arrangements made for blood transfusion if this exceeds 7.5% blood volume.

Table 12.1 Approximate peroperative fluid requirements compared with maintenance volumes

Age (years)	Volume (ml/kg/hour)	Maintenance volume (ml/kg/hour)
Birth to 3	2.75	6.3–4.25
3–5	2.5	3.75
5–9	2	3.75–3
9–13	1.75	3
Adult	1.5	2
	(as 0.18% saline/4.3% dextrose)	

Postoperative management

Restricted maintenance fluid (as for peroperative volumes) should be supplied for 24 hours, following which normal maintenance volumes may be given. It must be emphasized that abnormal losses occurring during and immediately after the operation must be replaced volume for volume with a suitable electrolyte content.

Complications

The foregoing sections assume that normal homeostatic mechanisms are present. If they are not, as in uncontrolled diabetes mellitus or uraemia then additional abnormal losses will have to be accounted for. The management of the diabetic child during surgery is described in Chapter 7.

Raised intracranial pressure

Head injuries, neurosurgery, meningitis and encephalitis are likely to cause a rise in intracranial pressure, and fluid administration should be judicious. The aim should be to provide a stable circulation with a urine output of 1 ml/kg/hour (with a minimum of 0.5 ml/kg/hour) and a plasma osmolality of 300–315 mmol/kg. This is done by restricting maintenance fluid to 50–60% of normal, usually given as 0.18% saline in 5% dextrose with potassium supplements. The electrolyte prescription may need to be varied in the light of abnormal losses, such as CSF drainage (replaced with 0.45% sodium chloride and dextrose) or diabetes insipidus. Continual reassessment is required in these patients as under-provision of fluids may lead to shock and renal impairment. Drug therapy should be given with care; sulphadiazine should not be given to patients on fluid restriction as crystalluria and acute renal failure may occur. The detailed monitoring and management of intracranial pressure is now recognized as an important function of paediatric intensive care, and compromise of the cerebral circulation and perfusion is now receiving as much attention as systemic circulatory failure.

13

The Newborn Infant

Just as the older child needs different management from the adult, so the newborn baby has different requirements from the child. Fluid intake is low in the first few days of life and the electrolyte requirements vary with gestational age.

Physiology

Renal bloodflow and glomerular filtration are low because the demands on the excretory function of the human kidney are small, especially when the infant is fed breast milk. A large part of the nutritional intake is used for growth so a correspondingly smaller amount is metabolized and excreted, therefore the infant kidney does not need to have the excretory capacity of the adult. The breast fed baby takes in sufficient water with solute to produce a hypotonic urine, and thus has a large reserve to accommodate abnormal fluid loss such as in diarrhoea. The baby fed on cow's milk does not take in so much water, its solute is less efficiently converted into growth and the urine is more concentrated. There is therefore less reserve to compensate for abnormal fluid loss.

Water

For the first 24–48 hours of life excretion of water is limited by the low GFR. (This is not the same as dilutional capacity; this is a renal tubular function which is normal in the newborn.) Therefore less exogenous fluid is needed immediately after birth, with the amount required gradually increasing over the first week. The concentrating capacity of the neonatal kidney is less well developed, reaching a maximum of about 650 mmol/kg, whereas the minimum achieved by older children and adults is 800 mmol/kg and may extend to over 1200 mmol/kg. The kidney of a newborn infant is capable of adaptation and if high solute milks are consistently given the concentrating power will increase more rapidly.

Electrolytes

The most important ion to the baby is sodium; sodium handling by
the newborn (particularly preterm) differs from the older child in
two important ways. Firstly, the kidney of the preterm infant cannot
retain sodium as efficiently as does the older child, and hyponatraemia may occur in the low birth-weight preterm infant unless
adequate intake is supplied. This is why formula cow's milk feeds
have to be specially adapted for preterm infants, with a higher
sodium content than those milks designed for mature babies. These
are particularly useful if natriuretic drugs such as theophylline are
used. Secondly, and more importantly to the full-term baby, the low
GFR in the baby means that sodium will not be filtered so easily at
the glomerulus, and salt and water retention will readily occur if excess is given.

Acid/base balance

Just as sodium handling is different in infancy so is hydrogen ion
excretion. The combination of low GFR and tubular immaturity will
result in a limited excretion of an acid load.

Water and electrolyte requirements

Fluid and electrolyte imbalance should be managed according to
the customary calculation framework.

Maintenance:

volume	60–120 ml/kg for days 1–4
	150 ml/kg/24 hours by day 5–7
composition	Na^+ 2 mmol/kg/24 hours
	K^+ 2 mmol/kg/24 hours
	H^+ none in short term
	Ca^{++} none in short term
energy	5–10% dextrose

Abnormal maintenance: as indicated by clinical circumstances.
Deficit: as indicated by clinical circumstances.

  Electrolyte requirement in the first few days is very variable,
especially in the sick infant, and it is better to underestimate the
amount needed. The maintenance fluids may need to be increased if
the baby is nursed under a radiant heater, or decreased if urine

volume decreases during severe intercurrent illness with hyponatraemia. Crystalloid infusions should only be given for a few days or
as a supplement to some other feeding. If enteral nutrition is not
going to be practical, then intravenous feeding should be started according to the regimen described in Chapter 11.

Fluid therapy in the newborn infant is precarious; regular
clinical examination including weighing, measurement of plasma
electrolytes and scrutiny of charts is required. Underhydration
causes prolonged physiological jaundice, a depressed fontanelle
and reduced tissue perfusion, which is best seen in the skin but is
possibly more harmful in splanchnic capillaries and in the cerebral
and renal circulations. Underhydration can occur quickly and increased fluid volumes should be given. The 150 ml/kg/24 hours is
time-honoured but is a guideline only. Overhydration may occur
through miscalculation — particularly when flushing catheters — or
because of reduced requirements in the sick infant. The consequences are well known: fluid overload leading to congestive heart
failure, hypertension and the increased likelihood of a persistent patent ductus arteriosus. Treatment is by fluid and electrolyte restriction and diuretics.

Techniques of fluid administration

Peripheral veins in the scalp or limbs should be used. The site
should not be covered with plaster or dressings when a constant
volume pump is used, as extravasation may cause ischaemia and
necrosis of the skin. The umbilical vessels should be avoided.

Complications

Neonatal hypoglycaemia

Although the infant can withstand lower glucose levels than adults
and older children symptomatic hypoglycaemia is serious because
if untreated it can lead to permanent neurological and intellectual
disability. It is therefore an emergency requiring immediate treatment. Asymptomatic hypoglycaemia will not cause neurological
damage and treatment can be less immediate. The causes are shown
in Table 13.1.

Prevention

Early milk feeds should be given to infants at particular risk of developing hypoglycaemia.

Diagnosis

1   Screening: babies at risk from any condition in Table 13.1 should be screened 4–12 hourly for 48 hours using a stix test (Dextrostix, BM-stix).
2   Babies with any symptom that is inexplicable should have a stix blood glucose test done. Note that stix tests must be done on stix whose shelf life has not expired and which have been kept in a cool place.

Table 13.1 Causes of neonatal hypoglycaemia (plasma glucose ⩽ 1.2 mmol/l)

> **1** Lack of glycogen:
> small-for-date infants
> preterm infants
> intrapartum anoxia
> any severe illness in mother or baby
> **2** Excess insulin:
> infants of diabetic mothers
> haemolytic disease of the newborn
> other rare syndromes
> **3** Others (rare):
> endocrine deficiency, e.g. adrenogenital
>   syndrome
> glycogen storage disease
> galactosaemia
> inborn errors of amino acid metabolism

Treatment

Asymptomatic hypoglycaemia: give the next milk feed immediately and check the blood glucose 1 hour later. If satisfactory, continue with normal feeding. If not, treat as symptomatic.

Symptomatic hypoglycaemia: a bolus dose of 5 ml/kg of 10% dextrose should be followed by an infusion of 2.5 ml/kg/hour of 10% dextrose. When feeding is re-established the infusion rate may be reduced provided that the blood glucose is acceptable and steady.

This reduction must be gradual to avoid rebound hypoglycaemia. Excessive infusion of glucose (e.g. > 5 ml/kg/hour of 10% dextrose) may cause hyperglycaemia, an osmotic diuresis and dehydration, so capillary blood glucose levels must be closely monitored.

Hypocalcaemia

The foetus has a higher plasma calcium than its mother. This suppresses foetal parathyroid function and allows a high plasma phosphate. After birth the calcium level quickly falls but the phosphate remains high because of: (1) delayed parathyroid hormone production; (2) the phosphate load of formula feeds; and (3) the low glomerular filtration rate. Other influences on plasma calcium levels (principally causing a fall) are hormones such as cortisol, drugs such as citrate in transfused blood, and acid/base balance. The level of ionized calcium determines whether symptoms occur, and this may vary with the blood pH — acidosis tending to raise the level of ionized calcium. Symptomatic neonatal hypocalcaemia (total plasma calcium < 1.5 mmol/l) causes neuromuscular irritability and convulsions. The causes are shown in Table 13.2.

Table 13.2   Causes of neonatal hypocalcaemia

Early
1 Secondary to any acute illness
2 Infants of diabetic mothers

Later
3 Phosphate-rich formula milk feeds (5–7 days; neonatal tetany)
4 Exchange transfusions
5 Absent parathyroids (DiGeorge syndrome)
6 Maternal factors:
hyperparathyroidism
vitamin D deficiency leading to secondary hyperparathyoidism

Treatment

Treatment is by intravenous 10% calcium gluconate 1 ml infused over 2 minutes. The hazards are: (1) bradycardia, so an ECG should be monitored; and (2) subcutaneous extravasation. This infusion should be followed by oral 10% calcium gluconate 2 ml before feeds for 24 hours; rarely a continuous intravenous infusion is required. Alternative, but less widely used, treatments are phosphate binders, such as aluminium hydroxide, or vitamin D. Failure of the treatment may result from accompanying hypomagnesaemia.

Hypomagnesaemia

Hypomagnesaemia (plasma level < 0.75 mmol/l) maybe caused by similar conditions as those predisposing to hypocalcaemia. Treatment is magnesium sulphate 50% 0.1 ml/kg (= 0.15 mmol/kg) given orally or parenterally.

14

The Burned Child

General

Children under the age of 14 years account for 30–50% of admissions to burn units. Burn injuries are uncommon in children below the age of 9 months, but rise sharply in incidence between the ages of 1 and 3 years, and are particularly common in the second year of life. The majority of these injuries result from hot fluid scalds in the home, for example from kettles, tea pots, cups of tea and coffee, and less commonly from accidental falls into baths or sinks of hot water. Only a few will result from contact with bars of electric fires, electric irons and other non-fluid sources. Although the number of deep flame burns due to clothes igniting (especially nightdresses) have been reduced in the last 15 years as a consequence of both improved clothing legislation and changes in the pattern of domestic heating appliances, injuries are still unacceptably frequent. A small proportion of childhood burns and scalds will result from non-accidental injury, which should always be suspected if the pattern of injury is unusual or when the history of injury is at variance with the distribution of the burn.

Physiology

Scalds and flame burns to the skin cause increased capillary permeability and a resultant loss of protein-rich fluid from the intravascular compartment into the interstitial tissues. When the area of skin affected exceeds 10–12% of the body surface area (BSA) of a child the risk of developing clinically significant hypovolaemia exists. Because of the limited ability of a child to compensate for such fluid loss by the oral route alone, childhood burns over 10% BSA may well require additional intravenous fluid replacement.

Fluid assessment

It is generally accepted that intravenous fluid therapy in a burned child should be related to the percentage of body surface area (%

BSA) burned. A practical approach in assessing the area is to consider the surface area of the palm of the patient's hand (including the fingers) as 1% BSA, and to calculate the percentage of the burn from how many times the patient's palm will cover the burned area. When assessing the total BSA burned, areas of erythema alone should not be included as this is likely to overestimate the probable fluid requirements. If erythematous areas subsequently blister an adjustment to the fluid need calculation can be made. Children aged less than 5 years have a large surface area relative to body weight, the head and neck representing twice the proportion of BSA which this region represents in the adult (Table 14.1). These patients exhibit much greater variation in fluid needs than do older children or adults.

Table 14.1 Differing proportions (given as percentage of total BSA) for body surface area with age

Site	Age (years)				
	1	3	5	10	adult
Head and neck	20	18	16	11	9
Trunk	37	37	37	36	36
Upper limbs	16	16	16	17	18
Lower limbs	27	29	31	36	36
Perineum	1	1	1	1	1

Various formulae have been developed to estimate the likely amount of intravenous fluids needed, but it is important that such calculations are considered simply as an initial guide and that the fluid actually administered relates to the clinical response of the child. Burned children are often admitted to hospital late in the day. Since the first 12 hours following a burn is the period of maximum fluid loss, a burn of 10–12% BSA, which might otherwise have been managed with oral fluids alone by day, may be more safely managed overnight by setting up an intravenous infusion rather than by intermittent oral fluids. Children may sustain burns while already ill from some other cause (e.g. respiratory tract infections or gastroenteritis) and these pre-existing conditions will further increase fluid resuscitation requirements, as well as complicating the assessment of clinical response.

Treatment

Most burned children admitted to hospital have burns affecting less than 10% BSA. Accurate initial assessment of the extent of the burn is essential and clothing should be removed to allow this. It is highly desirable to reassure both the patient and parents concerning the extent of injury and the treatment to be given.

Active cooling of a major burn wound is best avoided because of the high risk of hypothermia. The burn wound should simply be covered with paraffin gauze and wrapped in dressing gauze. Blankets should then cover the child to limit heat loss since the burned area will lose heat (and water) at a rate much higher than for undamaged skin.

Minor burns

Treatment will depend on the age of the child and the home circumstances. If in doubt about the quality of observation or treatment then it is better to admit the child to hospital. Here, providing the burn is less than 10% BSA oral fluid therapy should suffice, giving maintenance fluid and electrolyte requirements plus 5–15% in the first 24 hours. Local treatment and analgesia will be needed and the urine output, blood pressure and pulse must be monitored.

Severe burns

Treatment at district hospital

If the burn appears to exceed 10% BSA a peripheral intravenous line should be established. It will be advantageous if this stage of the resuscitation process is started after initial telephone consultation with the burn unit to which the child is to be referred. Since the fluid lost from the burn area is protein-rich and very similar in composition to plasma, it should be replaced with colloid (freeze-dried plasma or plasma protein fraction). The most convenient colloid formula to use is that introduced by Muir and Barclay, which uses % BSA burn and body weight to calculate the likely intravenous colloid requirement in the periods of 4, 4, 4, 6, 6 and 12 hours postburn. It must be emphasized that all fluid requirement calculations are timed from the onset of burn injury and not from the time of admission to hospital. The initial intravenous fluid calculation of the Muir and Barclay formula is made according to: intravenous colloid

requirement (ml) for each post-burn period = % BSA burn × body
weight (kg)/2. This is equivalent to 2.5 ml colloid/kg/% BSA burn/24
hours post-burn.

Powerful (opiate) analgesia is rarely indicated at this stage of
management. It is also unlikely at this stage that respiratory problems will be evident, but the presence of soot in the nostrils should
be noted. A history of a flame burn in an enclosed space provides
the best warning of possible pulmonary problems later. Whilst such
pulmonary complications may require management by later endotracheal intubation and ventilation, this is rarely required in the
first few hours. With a secure intravenous line in position and the
child well wrapped, transfer to the nearest burn unit may now be
undertaken. Antitetanus prophylaxis should be given.

Treatment at burn unit

On arrival the extent and probable depth of the burn should be
reassessed. The commonest finding is that the size of the burn has
been overestimated, and correct assessment at this stage will allow
an early adjustment to be made in fluid calculations. Wound swabs
are taken on admission, and if haemolytic streptococci are grown
the patient is isolated and treated with penicillin. Haemolytic strep-
tococcal infections may prevent the take of skin grafts.

At the burn unit the child should be nursed in a warm to hot environment (25–30°C) to limit heat and water loss from the burn surface. By promoting peripheral vasodilatation this warm environment should limit any rise in either core temperature or blood
pressure — both of which cause convulsions in the burned child.
Early adequate fluid replacement should also prevent the complication of hypovolaemia and its consequences of organ failure and
hyperpyrexia. In addition to intravenous colloid, oral maintenance
fluids can be given as vomiting should be uncommon unless opiate
analgesics have been given. However, electrolyte-free solutions
should be administered with care, giving small amounts intermit-
tently as hyponatraemia (plasma sodium < 125 mmol/l) may also be
associated with convulsions during burn resuscitation.

Response to administered resuscitation fluids should be judged
primarily on clinical grounds — cerebral state, peripheral skin circulation, and pulse and respiration rates. In addition 4-hourly
measurements of the packed cell volume (haematocrit) may help in
determining the degree of haemoconcentration. A rising haema-

tocrit will usually indicate the need for an increase in the rate of plasma infusion. In the more severe burns a bladder catheter will be inserted and hourly urine output measurements made (a urine volume of 1 ml/kg/hour is often cited as an adequate output). Perhaps more important than hourly urine volume measurements are assessments of 24-hourly urine sodium, potassium, osmolality, urea and creatinine output, since renal failure following burn injury may be non-oliguric. The observation and comparison of peripheral temperature and core temperature is a useful technique in gauging the adequacy of intravenous fluid resuscitation, with the peripheral temperature kept as close as possible to the core temperature.

Full-thickness circumferential burns of the chest or limbs and digits should be released by making an incision down to the fat (escharotomy) in order to limit any risk of restriction of chest movements and to prevent any compromise of circulation to the extremities — especially digits. Although badly burned patients develop anaemia (partly due to red cell destruction by haemolysis and partly to bleeding from the burn surface, particularly if escharotomies have been performed) blood transfusion is rarely required during the initial resuscitation phase when haemoconcentration is already a problem.

Associated inhalation injury may alter fluid requirements and this is particularly true if the patient requires mechanical ventilation. Mechanical ventilation will be required if oxygen therapy (with or without endotracheal intubation) fails to maintain adequate arterial oxygen saturation. If there is any significant degree of parenchymal pulmonary damage there will be a very real risk of fluid therapy exacerbating pulmonary oedema, and in these patients fluid therapy should be monitored carefully. However, because of the dangers of septicaemia in burn-injured patients central venous lines and cardiac output measurements (Swan–Ganz catheters) should probably be avoided.

The initial dressing to the burn will probably be silver sulphadiazine cream, aimed at limiting bacterial growth on the burn surface. After the initial 36–48 hours of intensive fluid replacement the need for supplementary energy intake takes priority (420 J/kg/24 hours) and a fine-bore nasogastric tube is used if necessary. Such levels of energy intake are vital if the intense catabolism of the burn injury is to be countered.

The commonest reason for patients to fail to respond to fluid resuscitation after burn injury is that there has been a delay of several hours between the injury and the commencement of fluid replacement. Patients may appear deceptively well for the first 4–6 hours post-burn whilst the activation of the sympathetic nervous system compensates for increasing fluid loss by vasoconstriction. However, once this response becomes inadequate to compensate for continuing hypovolaemia signs of shock will intervene — and such shock may be irreversible.

15

Blood and Blood Product Transfusions

Children may need infusion of blood products for many different reasons. Unless there is immediate threat to life it is preferable to make a diagnosis (or obtain samples of blood to allow a diagnosis to be made) before administering blood. Transfusion products are shown in Table 15.1.

Technique

The blood should be administered with the minimum of delay to avoid bacterial contamination or degradation of the blood product. Great care should be taken to avoid transfusion of the wrong blood. The hospital procedure for patient identification should be followed scrupulously, both in obtaining the original sample for cross-matching (and, in the case of the newborn, a sample from the mother) and completing the request form, and in the checking of the blood pack with the patient's name and number before giving the blood. If there is any doubt check with the laboratory.

The infusion line should be primed with 0.9% saline because dextrose solutions may haemolyze red cells: the intravenous, not arterial, route should be used.

Complications

The important complications are fluid overload and transfusion reactions.

1 Fluid overload. This will inevitably occur if infusion is too hasty; 5 ml/kg/hour is adequate for most clinical conditions.

2 Transfusion reactions. The commonest are febrile episodes with skin rashes, but occasionally anaphylaxis occurs. They can be managed with antihistamines and antipyretics and transfusion may continue with care. If more severe reactions occur future transfusion policy should be discussed with medical staff of the blood transfusion centre.

Another, more serious, reaction is that which occurs following infusion of mismatched blood or, rarely, plasma with high anti-A or

131

Table 15.1 Transfusion products

Product	Indication	Amount and comments
Whole blood	Acute blood loss	Volume for volume blood loss. Massive transfusions will require supplemental platelets and fresh frozen plasma. 10% calcium gluconate 0.15 ml/kg required to prevent citrate coagulopathy. Watch plasma K^+
Packed cells prepared by removing 66% of the citrated plasma; PCV $\simeq$ 60, Hb $\simeq$ 22 g	Non-urgent replacement of red cell mass	10 ml/kg will raise Hb by c. 3 g/dl
Human plasma protein fraction (HPPF): albumin 40 g/l, Na 130–160 mmol/l, K < 2 mmol/l; no clotting factors	Volume replacement, burns	10–20 ml/kg
Fresh frozen plasma (all coagulation factors)	Multiple coagulation defects	10–15 ml/kg
Platelets	Platelet depletion with symptoms, e.g. mucosal bleeding	1 unit/7 kg BW; do not attempt to raise platelet count to normal
Salt poor albumin	Symptomatic hypoalbuminaemia	1 g/kg; watch for fluid overload. Use with diuretic
Cryoprecipitate	Depletion of factor VIII	1 unit/7 kg BW will raise factor VIII level to 25%

anti-B haemagglutinins. Fever, rigor, and back and abdominal pain preceed haemoglobinuria. The transfusion must cease and the blood pack returned to the laboratory with a blood specimen from the patient. Liberal fluids and diuretics should be given to maintain a urine output, but oliguric renal failure should be anticipated and treated where necessary.

In the long term hepatitis may be caused by blood transfusions, either carrying hepatitis B or some other virus such as cytomegalovirus. The acquired immune deficiency syndrome (AIDS) is a recently recognized risk. These events are becoming less common with careful donor selection and serological testing. Children who receive repeated transfusions for haemoglobinopathies will develop iron overload unless some chelation programme is started.

Further Reading

Finberg, L., Karvath, R. E. and Fleischman, A. R. 1982 *Water and Electrolytes in Pediatrics*, W. B. Saunders, Philadelphia.

Willatts, S. M. 1982. *Lecture Notes on Fluid and Electrolyte Balance*. Blackwell Scientific Publications, Oxford.

Winters, R. W. (ed) 1973. *The Body Fluids in Pediatrics*. Little, Brown & Co., Boston.

Winters, R. W. 1982. *Principles of Pediatric Fluid Therapy*. Little, Brown & Co. Boston.

List of Abbreviations

ADH	antidiuretic hormone		Hb	haemoglobin
AIDS	acquired immune deficiency syndrome		HD	haemodialysis
			HHb	reduced haemoglobin
ARF	acute renal failure		HPPF	human plasma protein fraction
ATP	adenosine triphosphate			
BSA	body surface area		ICF	intracellular fluid
BW	body weight		IF	interstitial fluid
CA	carbonic anhydrase		i.v.	intravenous(ly)
CMP	cow's milk protein		IWL	insensible water loss
CRF	chronic renal failure		ORS	oral rehydration salts
CSF	cerebrospinal fluid		PD	peritoneal dialysis
CVP	central venous pressure		PV	plasma volume
ECF	extracellular fluid		SIADH	syndrome of inappropriate antidiuretic hormone
ECG	electrocardiograph			
ECV	extracellular volume			
GFR	glomerular filtration rate		TBW	total body water

Index

Page references in italic refer to figures and/or tables.